# #STRONGGIRL

# #STRONGGIRL

## 20-MINUTE WORKOUTS AND QUICK MEALS

TO KEEP YOU
## LEAN,
## TRIM,
## AND
## POWERFUL

PLAIN SIGHT PUBLISHING
AN IMPRINT OF CEDAR FORT, INC. • SPRINGVILLE, UT

# ALI HOLMAN

ISBN: 978-1-4621-1810-6

Published by Plain Sight Publishing, an imprint of Cedar Fort, Inc.,
2373 W. 700 S., Springville, UT 84663
Distributed by Cedar Fort, Inc., www.cedarfort.com

LIBRARY OF CONGRESS CATALOGING-IN-PUBLICATION DATA
Holman, Ali, 1973- author.
#StrongGirl : 20-minute workouts and quick meals to keep you lean, trim, and powerful / Ali Holman.
    pages cm
Includes bibliographical references.
ISBN 978-1-4621-1810-6 (layflat binding : alk. paper)
1. Physical fitness--Handbooks, manuals, etc. 2. Exercise for women. 3. Physical fitness--Nutritional aspects. I. Title.
GV436.H55 2015
613.7--dc23
                        2015032921

Cover and page design by Lauren Error
Cover design © 2015 by Lyle Mortimer
Edited by Eileen Leavitt

Printed in the United States of America

10  9  8  7  6  5  4  3  2  1

Printed on acid-free paper

*dedication*

I DEDICATE THIS BOOK TO MY TWO FAVORITE #STRONGGIRLS: AVA & DEMI. BEING YOUR MOM WILL ALWAYS BE THE BEST THING THAT HAS EVER HAPPENED TO ME. I LOVE YOU, I AM PROUD OF YOU, AND I ENCOURAGE YOU TO LIVE YOUR LIFE WITH STRENGTH AND FAITH.

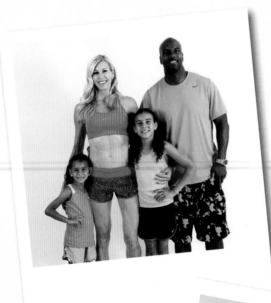

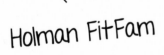

Holman FitFam

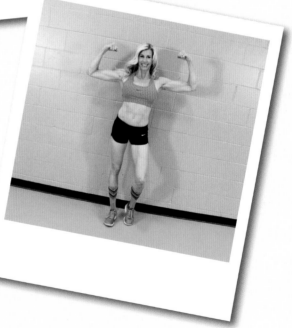

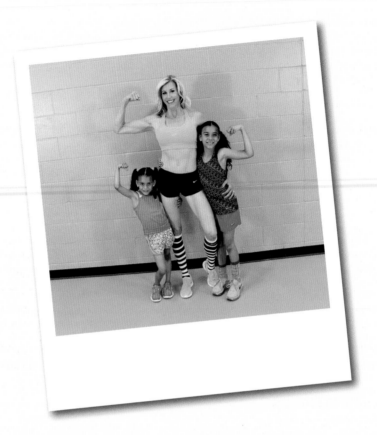

I REALLY STARTED TO THINK ABOUT THE WORD *SKINNY*, AND YOU KNOW THE FIRST THING THAT CAME TO MY MIND? **WEAK.**

Okay, I know what you might be thinking: *You're a fitness expert. You're a personal trainer. You are a nutrition magician.* (Or has that gone too far?) *Being "fit" is easy for you.*

The truth is, at the end of the day I am a mom. My kids don't care if I was on TV talking about the best exercises for your butt hours earlier. We have homework, we have tantrums, we have picky eaters, we have little feet following me to the bathroom, and we have chaos!

One of the hardest parts of parenting is worrying about your kids. With the childhood obesity rate skyrocketing, add weight and physical fitness to the list of concerns you grapple with not just for your kids, but also for yourself and your spouse.

I was a trainer long before I had kids and admittedly didn't "get it" until I did. I would wonder why clients couldn't just "find the time" to work out. Why couldn't they get their kids moving and just turn off the TV? Why couldn't they just tell their husbands to get up and work out with them? Then I married and had children, and reality hit me. Amidst a busy career and new marriage, finding time was tough. We celebrated our one-year anniversary with a newborn baby, and I remember insisting we go to a restaurant because it was our anniversary, hoping my daughter would stay asleep . . . and then leaving before our food arrived because we had a diaper blowout. Oh yeah. Reality hit us *hard*. Add kid number two, a TV career, a family online training business, three crazy dogs, and our nonstop life, and we are knee-deep in reality, baby.

This reality truly lead to my "aha" moment. I wasn't just placed in this position to help people get rock hard abs (although that is a huge bonus!); my personal mission became showing busy families like mine how to embrace fitness. I have met countless families that "have it together": perfect house, nice cars, love and support, and the list goes on. But the one issue they can't seem to get a handle on is health and fitness. Why is that? What I have discovered is that the central reason families seem to fight a losing battle against fitness and healthy living, despite understanding how important it is, is a matter of psychology. Parents are dealing with the same body issues, food issues, and emotional insecurities that they had when they were fourteen. Fast-forward twenty or thirty years, and they are now parents and successful adults, but they still have not found success with health and fitness. Frustrating, right?

Many years ago, I coined the term *StrongGirl*. I did this because I was having my first daughter, and for the first time in my life, I *really* thought about the mental dialogue women have and also project in speaking their goals: "Look at you! You look great—so skinny," "I just want skinny thighs," and "She is so skinny, I hate her." You get the idea. I really started to think about the word *skinny*, and you know the first thing that came to my mind? *Weak.* When I think of a skinny woman, I don't automatically think *strong.* So that's when I had the idea. Instead of claiming the "skinny" title, I was going to own the "StrongGirl" title. That image projects strength, power, sexiness, confidence, and independence. Isn't that what I wanted my daughter and me to be? The answer was a resounding yes! From that point on, I would correct people when they would tell me they wanted to lose weight. I would point out that if they switched their goals to getting strong, the inches would fall off, and their confidence would soar. Who doesn't want to feel like they could conquer the world and kick a few butts?

I challenge you to embrace your inner #StrongGirl. There a few steps you can take to find her:

## 1. *Look in the mirror every day and say to yourself, "You are STRONG."*

I know it sounds crazy, but I do this every time I go into the bathroom. I look myself in the eye and remind myself that I am strong. When I am a guest at someone's house, they might think I am crazy talking to myself in the bathroom, but I know they also think I'm strong! Whether said aloud or even screamed in your head, words have power.

Think of this: Have you ever met a woman who is drop-dead gorgeous but always points out her own flaws? You are baffled—how in the world does she not see in herself what others see in her? But then it dawns on you—someone either in her childhood or in a relationship told her those things (probably repeatedly), and guess what—now she believes them. If you hear, "you are selfish" ten times, on the eleventh time you won't have to hear it because you will already believe it. Hearing, "Those pants are just not flattering on body types like ours" lingers in the head for much longer than it deserves and will haunt you for years in a dressing room. By telling yourself you are strong, you will rise to the occasion. It may take some weeks, but before you know it, this new truth will become your inner mantra. And if you think your kids don't watch these power words and eventually emulate them, think again.

## 2. *Surround yourself with StrongGirls.*

As women, we sometimes shy away from the other women who seem to have it all together. It's not because we don't like them, but sometimes we feel it highlights what we think we are not. StrongGirls have this problem sometimes. Whether it is because of the StrongGirl's confidence, muscles, or dedication to treat her body like a prized possession, other women often assume that a StrongGirl won't have time for them. Not true! Seek out these StrongGirls. Ask one of them if she would be willing to be your accountability partner. Share your journey with her. She has been on that exact same road and knows the directions well. Use her as a resource rather than being intimidated by her.

### 3. *Find her in your kids.*

Have kids? Well, then welcome to the #StrongGirl club. Give yourself more credit! Look at what your body did! Not only is pregnancy is beautiful, but it also requires a tremendous amount of strength. Think you don't have enough dedication to stick to a workout program? Well, look at your dedication to your family. They are getting the best of you, and you are getting the scraps. The problem with that formula is that your best is often struggling. The true key to a StrongMom is a woman who recognizes she has to take care of her health and wellness in order to be the best for herself and her family. This is not selfish. In fact, it's imperative. A healthy, strong, energetic mom will run circles around a tired, weak, ailment-ridden mom any day. Do it for you, and everyone else will benefit.

### 4. *Find a program you can weave into your busiest day.*

One of my biggest pet peeves about New Year's resolutions is there is a rumor that on January 1, we all will wake up with an extra hour to exercise. NOT! That is why the typical fitness New Year's resolution dies a quick death after an average of eight days. Here is what I tell my clients and why we created our Under 20-Minute Daily Online Core-Camper.com workouts. Think of your busiest day. I mean the one with a school conference, sick kid, forgetful husband, and meetings galore, and then choose the workout program that will fit into that day. This is why we created our Under 20-Minute Daily Online CoreCamper.com workouts. If you are looking for an excuse to not work out and you are a mom, chances are you can find one—and a good one at that. But who are you really cheating? Not only will a quick workout give you some perspective on the day, it will also reduce stress and boost confidence—not to mention burn some fat!

## SO WHAT ABOUT MY FAMILY?

My belief is that the first thing you have to do is make fitness a family value. Just as you are raising your kids to go to church regularly, to volunteer, or to stick to their promises—you also raise them to understand that the body they have is the only body they get. Abusing your body, not exercising, and using food as a reward system are just a few ways moms set the tone early on. These habits teach our children to devalue a healthy body.

Committing to be fit together as a family is all about baby steps, and in this book, I am going to give you the tools to start moving forward. Being fit is not an exclusive club, it's not a path of punishment, and it is not something you should dread. My goal is to show you how we have done it as a family and how you can too!

# WHAT DOES "FIT" REALLY MEAN?

Your mind might immediately go to bulging muscles and ripped abs, but being fit really starts from within. I often compare it to those who choose to get sober. This is a process that takes steps, daily recommitment, and surrounding yourself with people who support your endeavor. I often meet people who are almost embarrassed to announce that they are embarking on a healthy journey. I once had a client tell me, "I'm not even going to tell my husband because if I fail, he will say 'I told you so.'" My response to her was for her to consider the sentence she had just spoken to me. *If I fail* is a phrase that holds a lot of power. It sets the stage for failure and, in fact, welcomes it into the room with open arms.

When you and your family make the decision to embark on a journey of health and fitness, talk about how you are going to talk about it. I even encourage people to write down Power Phrases and put them up where they are visible in their homes. You will find some of these Power Phrases scattered throughout the book:

1.  FITNESS IS MY LIFESTYLE.

2.  EATING CLEAN FEELS AMAZING.

3.  I EAT HEALTHY TO FUEL MY BODY.

4.  THIS IS THE ONLY BODY I HAVE, AND I WILL TREAT IT ACCORDINGLY.

5.  I WILL NOT "TREAT MYSELF" WITH FOOD.

6.  I AM STRONG AND UNIQUE.

7.  I WILL NOT COMPARE MYSELF TO OTHERS.

8.  I WANT TO LIVE A LONG AND HEALTHY LIFE.

9.  I WILL TREAT A SETBACK AS A COMEBACK.

10. WHAT I AM DOING TODAY WILL HELP ME IN ONE, TEN, AND TWENTY YEARS FROM NOW.

Don't you just *feel* better reading these phrases? Now imagine them as a part of your inner mantra. This can be who you are not only as a mom but also as an entire family. It is yours to claim.

# "MOM! MOM! MOM! MOM! MOM! . . . DAD! WHERE'S MOM?!"

I don't know about you, but in my family, as Mom I often set the tone. My kids know it too. They don't even bother to ask my husband anymore when we are leaving for an event or where we are going out to dinner. "I don't know. Ask Mom" is what I usually hear muffled from upstairs when my kids get tired of trying to find me. (And I admit it—sometimes I *am* hiding from them!)

But what if we took that influence as Mom and used our powers for good? We set the tone for our household. What about setting the tone for making fitness a priority? What about shopping for healthy foods and seeking information on how to better take care of our bodies? Don't you think our kids would follow that lead?

My nine-year-old surprised me the other day. For years, I have fixed her naturally curly hair every morning, sometimes causing tears and, more recently, lots of eye rolling. I never thought she paid attention and, in fact, thought she loathed any hair fixing of any sort. The other day, she had a friend over, and she and asked if she could fix the friend's hair. I could hear them from the other room, and my daughter, Ava, was even using my lines: "I am going to use this comb to make a straight part—it might hurt a little bit, but I will try and be gentle. . . ." It dawned on me that—*hallelujah!*—she actually *is* listening to me when she is acting like what I am doing is the most inconvenient thing in the world!

Nutrition and exercise are no different. I have actually found my girls creating and writing down workouts to do together. They are ten and five. I know what you are thinking: *You probably make them do that because you are a fitness expert.* But the answer is no! I never push fitness and nutrition on my kids. Instead, I model it. And it works. I hear them in their playroom saying, "Keep your butt down on that plank!" and "twenty seconds left! We can do this!" and then they give each other high fives when they are done.

Don't believe me? Try it. Pull out your exercise mat and work out in front of your kids. Chances are if they don't drop down and try the moves right then, you will catch them trying it in their room later. Modeling is nothing new in parenting, but why do we assume it doesn't include healthy eating and fitness?

Make the decision to use that leadership role in your family to incorporate health. It might just be one of the best uses of power ever known to mankind.

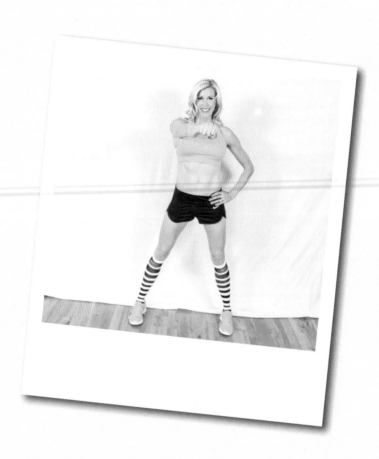

THAT MEANS NO BABYSITTER, NO GERMY GYM DAY CARES,
NO MOMMY GUILT, AND MAJOR RESULTS IN A
**SHORT AMOUNT OF TIME.**

# CHAPTERONE
## Work Out *Smarter*, Not Longer

Motherhood is an amazing gift, but it can also hit your body like a ton of bricks. Having intentions of working out after you have a baby and finding the time and energy to really do it are two separate things. Whether you are sleep-deprived, are nursing, have a cranky baby, or are a cranky mommy—time is one of the hardest things to find with kids.

## SCHEDULE TIME FOR YOU

Between dentist appointments, school conferences, office meetings, date nights, and sporting events, most of us are pretty on the ball with keeping our commitments and showing up. But what about making time for you? The "I don't have time" excuse sneaks into a workout plan quite often, and my first suggestion is to not "try" to fit it in—but rather to schedule it. We innately are doers. Doesn't it feel great to make a list and check things off?

I suggest using the same strategy when it comes to your workouts. Make them a non-negotiable item and keep them as high on the priority list as one of your kids' events or obligations. Here are a few easy ways to visualize your goals and track your progress:

### *The Calendar Method*

I suggest that instead of making monthly promises and goals with yourself, make weekly short-term goals instead. Box out a week on your calendar with a colored marker. (Yes, I'm asking you to go old-school and print out an actual calendar sheet!) You'll want five out of seven days to have check marks on them. Those check marks represent your 20-minute workout done. If you get to Wednesday and see that you are lacking check marks, it's time to kick it into high gear. Have a reward for yourself each week (be sure you choose a reward that is not food related) if you reach that goal. Gift yourself a pedicure, a hot bath, a new pair of workout shoes, a download of a new song, or coffee at your favorite spot. The idea is the splurge is just for you and a time for you to pause and say, "Hey, I did it!" Celebrate your weekly accomplishments, and if you have a bad week, your new week is just around the corner!

### *The Rock Method*

I love this visualization method because it works. Take two bowls and write, "Workouts To Do" on one and "Workouts DONE!" on the other. Put five rocks in the "To Do" bowl at the beginning of the week. After each workout is completed, move a rock over. It seems simple, but try it for a week, and you will see just how good it feels to have the "DONE" bowl full!

### *Lay It Out*

Every Sunday night, I lay out my workout clothes for my five "To Do" workouts for the week, all the way down to the headband and socks. I lay them across my closet floor so I have to see them, step over them, and be reminded by them every day. This saves time when you are ready to squeeze in a workout and is a great daily reminder. At the end of the week, you will have a cleared-off floor and a healthy body. It's a win-win!

PS: It also is great motivation to buy those cute workout clothes you've had your eye on!

## SMARTER, NOT LONGER

Research is a wonderful thing, and when it proves that the type of workout you do is more important than the amount of time you spend doing it, you want to give it a big kiss. Gone are the days of posting up on the elliptical machine for two hours to get a "good workout." The American College of Sports Medicine's (ACSM) Michael Bracko, EdD, FACSM, describes "HIIT" (high intensity interval training) exercises as providing similar benefits to endurance exercises but in a shorter time. Bracko's findings show that a person consumes more oxygen during HIIT than in slower, distance exercise, which can increase post-exercise metabolism. Research has shown one session of HIIT can burn calories for 1½ to 24 hours after exercise![1] Sign me up! In fact, I would venture to say they are *more* effective. By integrating interval training into your fitness routine—no matter what your starting fitness level—you don't plateau, you don't get bored, and your body does not adapt to one particular exercise.

So how effective is this? Consider this: A person running an approximate 8-minute mile will burn an average of about 150 calories in twenty minutes. While doing interval training, utilizing multiple muscle groups at once, the average calorie burn can double. Not only do you get a huge bang for your buck during your workout, but you also benefit from the "afterburn effect," which means your body continues to burn calories for hours after your interval training workout.

In this chapter, I want to show two amazing ways to fit in a 20-minute fitness routine that you can do at home or at the park with your family. That means no babysitter, no germy gym day cares, no mommy guilt, and major results in a short amount of time. When I developed my under 20-minute daily online training program, CoreCamper.com, I decided not only to maximize this "smarter, not longer" technique but also use "equipment" people already have.

For these workouts, we will use a simple water jug, step stool, pillowcase, towels, and paper plates—or play equipment that can be found at almost any park. Not only will these be the most effective workouts you will ever do, they will also be the most affordable and fun!

## "USE WHAT YOU'VE GOT" WORKOUT

Perform each exercise for 45 seconds with a 15 second rest. Go through the following list twice.

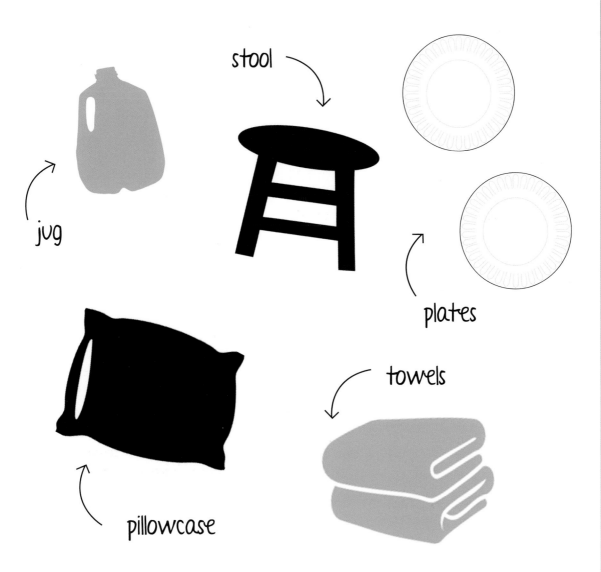

jug

stool

plates

towels

pillowcase

# **STEP STOOL** TOE TAP PUSH-UP

Put your feet on a step stool, and ensure your body is parallel to the ground. Pull your core in as you tap one foot off the stool toward your hand. Place that foot back on the stool, and then do a push-up. Repeat, alternating foot toe taps between push-ups.

STEP**1**

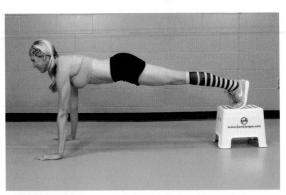

STEP**2**

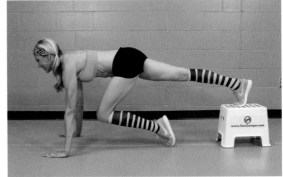

STEP**3**

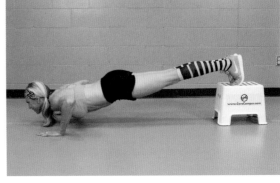

# TOWEL HILL CLIMBERS

Place your feet on hand towels on a slippery surface, such as wood, tile, or linoleum floors. Keep your body in a straight plank position (rear not in the air and hips not dropped). Start quickly "climbing," bringing feet forward toward your hands. Look forward, and make sure your back is flat and rear is down to keep your core engaged.

STEP **1**

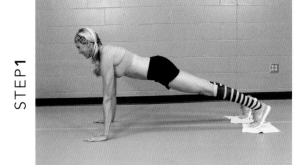

STEP **2**

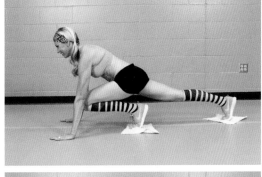

STEP **3**

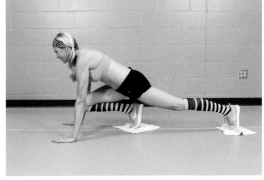

Sit, cross your feet, and keep them off the ground. Hold the jug and shift it side to side, on either side of the knees, allowing your core to twist as you face the jug on each side.

STEP **1**

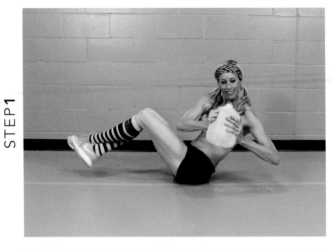

STEP **2**

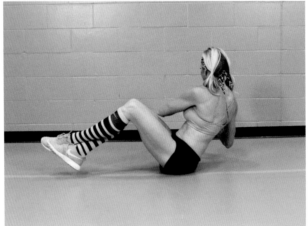

# **WATER JUG** BOAT SIDE-TO-SIDES

# PILLOWCASE LUNGE PRESS

Place water bottles or books in two pillowcases. Hold them down near your feet. Keeping your back straight, step forward in a lunge, ensuring your knee does not exceed past your shoelace. As you come up from your lunge, press your pillowcases overhead.

STEP **1**

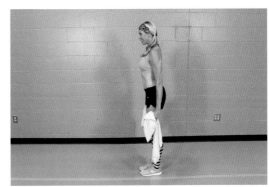

STEP **2**

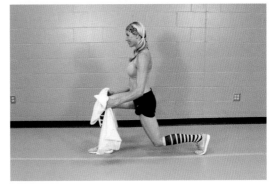

STEP **3**

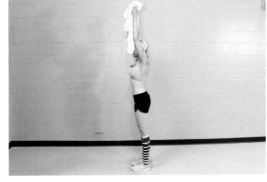

Place your hands on a stool, with your rear in the air and toes on the ground. In a quick motion, bring your heels to your rear and then land softly. Repeat without rest for entire interval.

STEP **1**

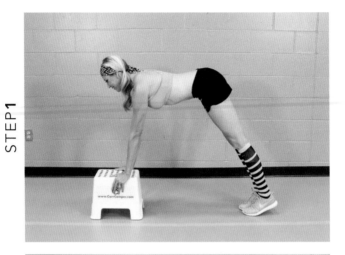

STEP **2**

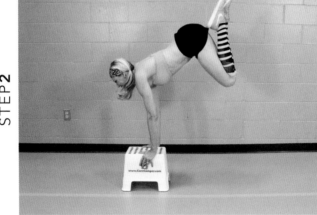

**STEP STOOL** DONKEY KICKS

Get in side plank position, with your right hand on ground, hips up, and legs straight. Your left leg will be in front of the right, with the left foot placed on a towel. Keeping your hips off ground and left hand on hip, make semicircles with the left foot (on towel). Repeat with the right foot forward.

STEP**1**

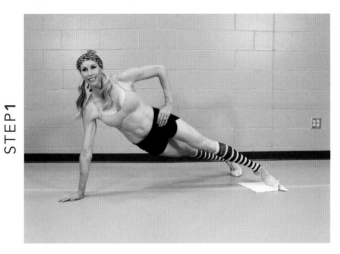

STEP**2**

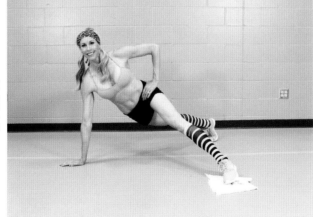

# **TOWEL** SIDE PLANK SEMICIRCLES

# PAPER PLATE PLANK PIKES

Get in elbow planks with your body parallel to ground. Place your feet on paper plates. Plates will slide on carpet, tile, wood, and linoleum. Slowly bring one knee into your chest, allowing the rear to raise. Place the foot back, and return the body to its parallel position. Repeat with the other foot. Continue for an entire interval.

STEP 1

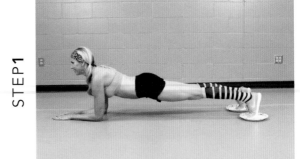

STEP 2

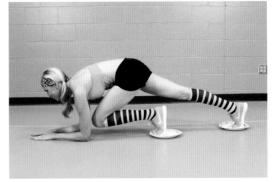

STEP 3

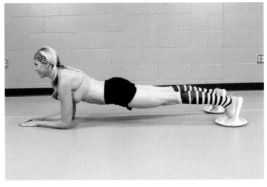

This is a great exercise that takes the place of a kettlebell swing. Hold the jug between the legs, looking forward, chest open, and knees bent. With a controlled upward swing, using your core as the primary force, drive the water jug toward the ceiling, stopping slightly above forehead level. Keep your arms straight, and do not hunch over. Continue this without rest for the entire interval.

STEP**1**

STEP**2**

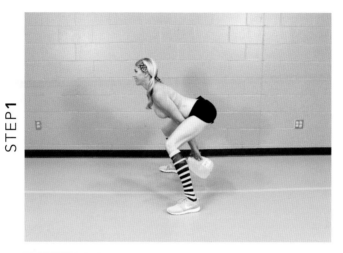

# **WATER JUG** SWING

# TOWEL HEEL PULL-INS

Get in a straight-arm reverse plank position, arms straight, hips raised, belly button facing the ceiling. Place your heels on a towel, and keep your hips squeezed up. Quickly pull your heels in, all while keeping your body in a straight position (strong core, no saggy bottom!)

STEP 1

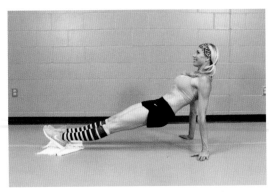

STEP 2

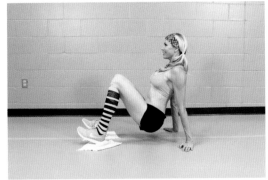

STEP 3

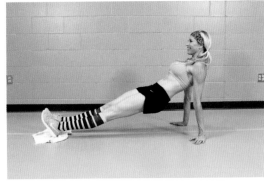

# SQUAT THRUST TO BELLY

You will torch the fat and work every muscle with this move. Place hands on the ground with body in a straight plank. Jump your feet up by your hands so you are in a crouching position. Jump feet back to straight plank and then slowly lower to belly, going down to the ground as one unit. Repeat.

STEP **1**

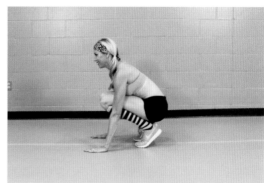

STEP **2**

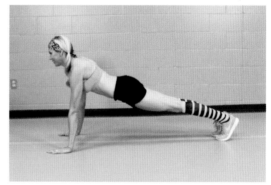

STEP **3**

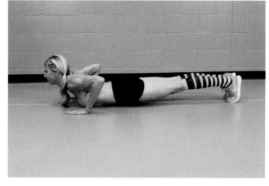

# CORECAMPER PARK WORKOUT

One of our favorite things to do as a family is to go to the park. The park is all about play, but who says you can't add some fitness fun to that playtime? The park is free and accessible to anyone, has amazing equipment you can use for workouts, and your kids will love that mom and dad are "playing" with them instead of looking at their phones and sitting on a bench!

### *How It's Done*

Find a park with swings, a slide, some sort of hanging bar, a step-up or stairs, a park bench, and monkey bars.

### *Time It Up*

To keep you on task, set a timer on your phone. (There are many free interval timer apps that will allow you to choose how many rounds and length of interval and rest time.)

Set your timer for 45 seconds of work, 20 seconds of rest (although you will use this "rest" time to get to the next station).

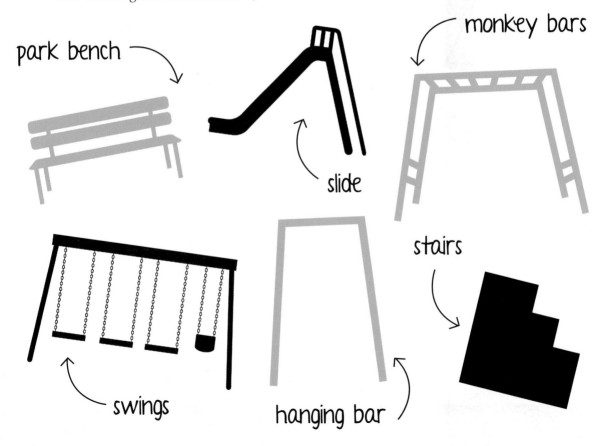

park bench

slide

monkey bars

stairs

swings

hanging bar

Where crunches work only about 25 percent of your core, engaging your core in a suspended straight-arm plank will work your abdominals, obliques, back, hips, and more. Think of your core as a large, thick belt wrapped around your waist—and all of it is fired up for this exercise.

Place your hands on a swing and your feet on the ground and hold a straight-arm plank. Your hands are directly under your shoulders, abs are pulled in, and body is in a straight, neutral position. Hold for 45 seconds.

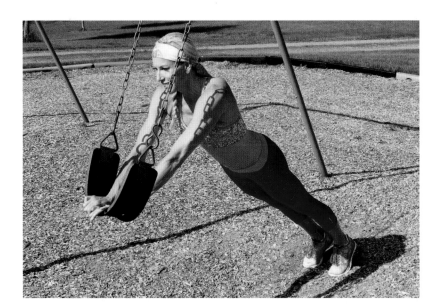

# **SWING** STRAIGHT-ARM PLANKS

Get your heart rate up and work your entire core, glutes, and upper body with this exercise.

Place your feet on the swing and hands on the ground. Keeping your hips engaged and neutral, bring your knees quickly to the chest and then place the feet back. Repeat for 45 seconds.

STEP**1**

STEP**2**

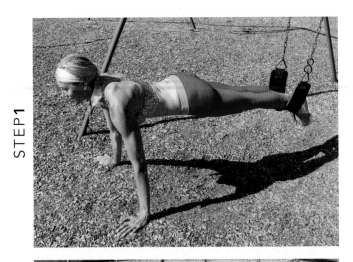

**SWING** SQUAT THRUSTS

# **SPIDERWOMAN** CRAWLS

Get your cardio and have some fun with this exercise. Crawl quickly up the slide, and then immediately slide down when you reach the top. Keep your body low, using your lower body to power up the slide quickly. Repeat for 45 seconds. This exercise works your entire lower body and gives you a great cardio workout.

**STEP 1**

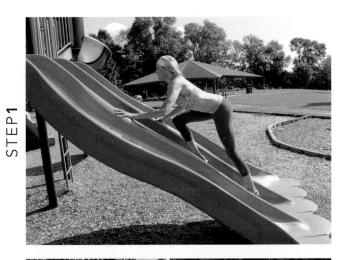

**STEP 2**

Place your feet at the end of the slide so they are slightly elevated off of the ground. Place your hands on ground and keep your body in a neutral, straight position. Repeat push-ups in this position for 45 seconds. This exercise works your core, chest, and upper body.

STEP1

STEP2

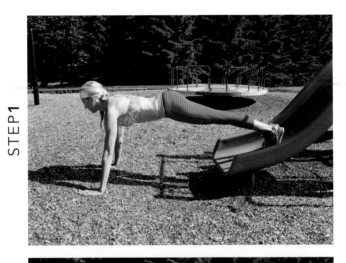

**SLIDE** ELEVATED PUSH-UPS

# **PULL-UP** TO THE BAR

It's not what you're thinking! Forward grip the bar and place your body in a diagonal position, with your heels on the ground and belly facing the bar. Keeping your body as a unit, row up, bringing chest to bar. Repeat for 45 seconds. This exercise works your entire core, upper body, and back.

STEP**1**

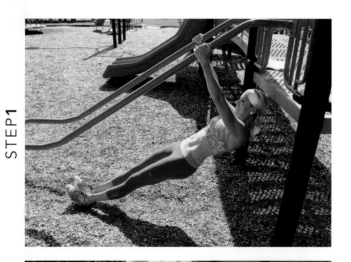

STEP**2**

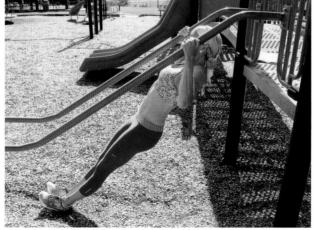

Hang from the bar with straight arms, heels on the ground. Slowly raise one straight leg off of the ground, squeezing your lower abs. Repeat, switching legs. This exercise focuses on your core, targeting lower abs.

STEP**1**

STEP**2**

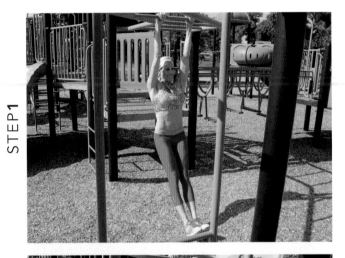

# **HANGING** STRAIGHT PLANK RAISES

# **QUICK** TOE TAPS

Elevate your heart rate with this low impact but powerful option. Place your hands on your hips, or place your hands above your head to engage the core, and quickly tap your foot on top of the steps or stairs, using a level that is challenging to you. Continue for 45 seconds. This exercise works your lower body and core and provides cardio.

STEP**1**

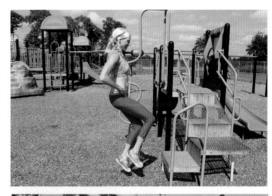

STEP**2**

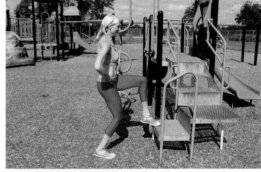

STEP**3**

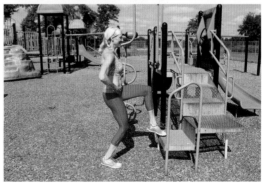

Crouch in front of a step with your knees bent and your hands on the step. Lunge back with one leg, driving your knee toward the ground. Repeat, switching feet each time, while looking forward. Keep your back in a flat, neutral position. Continue for 45 seconds. Step lunges work your lower body and increase cardio.

STEP**1**

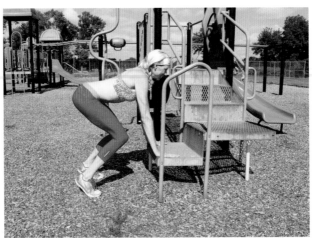

STEP**2**

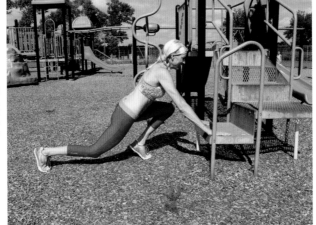

**STEP** LUNGES

# CRAB KICKS WITH TRICEP DIP

Place your hands on a bench, with your feet flat on the ground, bottom dropped. Quickly bring one leg up, crunching your nose toward that knee, tricep dipping at the same time. Repeat, switching feet.

Continue for 45 seconds. This works your core, upper body (primarily shoulders and triceps), and lower body, and it increases cardio.

STEP 1

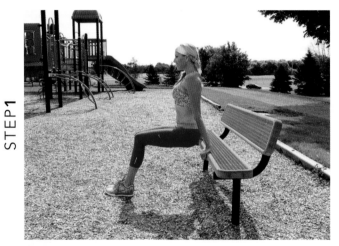

STEP 2

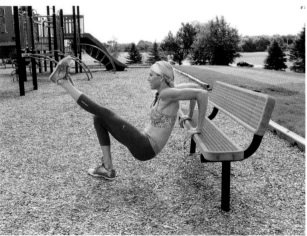

# **BENCH** LATERAL WALKS TO SQUAT THRUST

Place your feet on one end of a park bench, hands on the ground, and body in a neutral/straight position. Walk your hands and feet to other side of bench, keeping your rear down. At the end of the bench, jump your feet toward your hands, and then return to neutral position. Repeat for 45 seconds. This works your upper body, core, and lower body and is a good cardio exercise.

STEP**3**

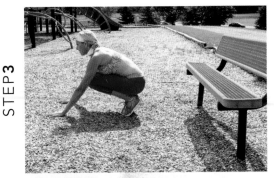

STEP**1**

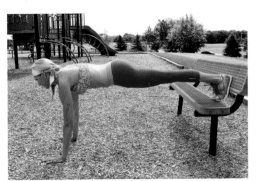

STEP**4**

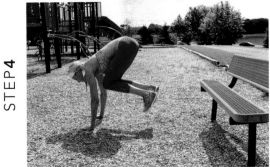

STEP**2**

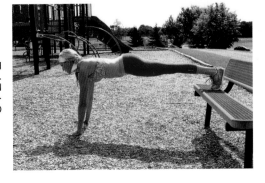

STEP**5**

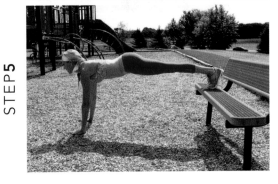

Hang from the monkey bars and run in place as quick as you can, bringing knees up to the chest, feet not touching ground. Repeat for 45 seconds. This exercise focuses on upper body, core, and cardio.

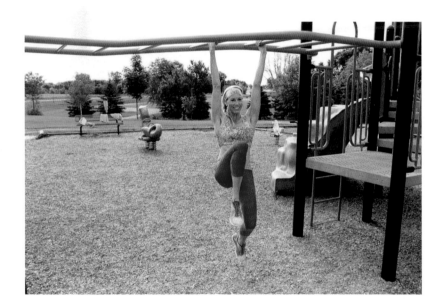

# **RUNNING** MAN/WOMAN

Starting at the end of the monkey bars, hop up and tap one rung. Repeat all the way down the bars, turn around, and repeat for 45 seconds. This exercise works the lower body and increases cardio.

STEP**1**

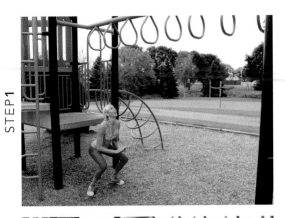

STEP**3**

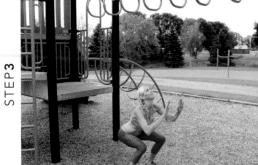

STEP**2**

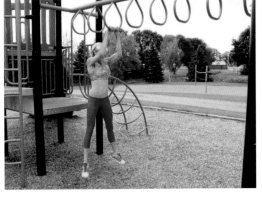

STEP**4**

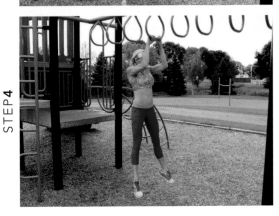

**MONKEY** HOPS

# Fitness is my lifestyle

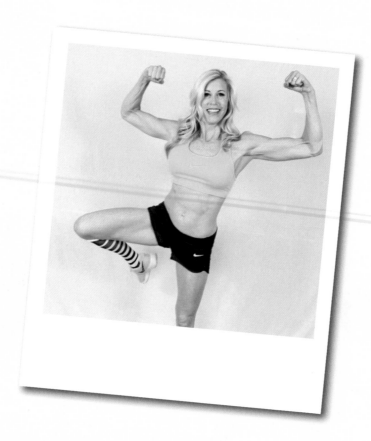

DON'T ANNOUNCE TO YOUR FAMILY THAT IT'S HEALTHY.
DON'T "SELL IT" AS HEALTHY. COME ON, PEOPLE!
**IT'S ALL ABOUT THE MARKETING!**

# CHAPTERTWO
## Sneaky Swaps & 20-Minute Easy, Healthy Recipes

Have you ever felt like a short-order cook but found yourself standing in your kitchen instead of a restaurant? Well, welcome to motherhood. I can't tell you how many moms I meet who are trying to eat healthy so they prepare one meal for themselves and a completely different meal for their family. But why? If you raise your kids on healthy foods, they may kick and scream initially, but it *will* become their norm. It also will more than likely be the path they follow as adults.

But here's the trick: Don't announce to your family that it's healthy. Don't "sell it" as healthy. Come on, people! It's all about the marketing!

I call this #SneakyHealthy. What they don't know won't hurt them. In fact, it will have the opposite effect. Making healthy eating a priority can be part of who you are as a family. And before you think it's too late—it's not. I encourage you to make the declaration, "We are a family that makes healthy eating a priority." It doesn't mean you never go for fast food. It doesn't mean you all eat salads. It means you weave healthy food into your life the majority of the time. And guess what, with these tricks, you'll love it.

Let's start with some simple recipe swaps you can make to cut calories, incorporate health, and improve nutrition without your family even noticing.

## SNEAKY SWAPS

### OTHER NUT BUTTERS INSTEAD OF PEANUT BUTTER

Almond butter has a nutritional advantage over peanut butter due to its vitamin E content. Almond butter contains approximately 4 milligrams of vitamin E per tablespoon—about 27 percent of your daily vitamin E requirements. Peanut butter contains just 1 milligram of vitamin E per 1-tablespoon serving.

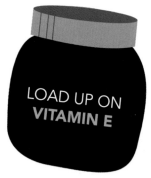

## AVOCADO INSTEAD OF MAYO

With almost half the calories and more fiber, healthy fats, and potassium—avocado is a great substitute for mayo on a sandwich. Avocados are lower in saturated fat than mayonnaise and contain "heart-healthy" monounsaturated fats. This kind of fat lowers cholesterol, decreases stomach pouch, and actually helps your heart. Plus, let's face it . . . avocados taste amazing!

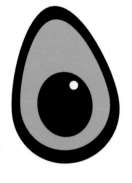

ADIOS TO 50% OF THE CALORIES

avocado

## INFUSED WATER INSTEAD OF JUICE

Parents often ask me what they can give their kids instead of juice. Try infused water! You save 3 teaspoons of sugar per serving, and your kids will still get that fruity fresh taste. Compare this: One glass of orange juice contains 240 calories and over 4 oranges. One large bottle of infused water with 3 slices of oranges boasts only 33 calories!

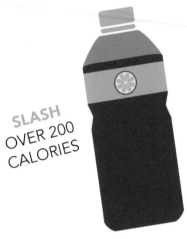

SLASH OVER 200 CALORIES

infused water

## GREEK YOGURT INSTEAD OF SOUR CREAM

Swap empty calories for 8 grams of protein per serving. Make sure to get the "plain" flavor—it is truly sour cream's doppelgänger! Same texture, same taste . . . but one cup of Greek yogurt has about 140 calories, whereas sour cream packs a 300-calorie punch.

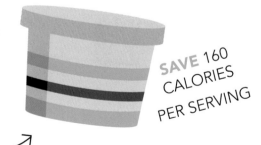

SAVE 160 CALORIES PER SERVING

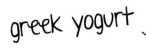

greek yogurt

## WHOLE GRAIN PASTA INSTEAD OF WHITE

The main difference between white and whole-wheat pasta lies in the processing. Whole-wheat pasta contains 3 parts of the grain—the bran (the grain's outer layer), the germ (the sprouting section of the seed), and the endosperm (the large starchy center). But during the refining process, the heat used to process the grain forces the nutrient-rich bran and germ out of the grain, leaving just the endosperm behind. While the stripped-down white stuff boasts a longer shelf life and is cheaper, it's considered nutritionally weaker.

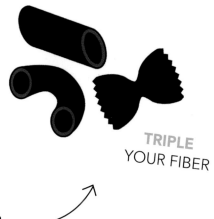

TRIPLE YOUR FIBER

whole grain pasta —

## STEEL-CUT OATMEAL INSTEAD OF GRANOLA

A half-cup cooked serving of steel-cut oats has just 150 calories, 2½ grams of fat, and 1 gram of sugar. If you sprinkle with cinnamon, you add zero calories and the perfect amount of flavor. Granola, on the other hand, is not as healthy as it looks. The same half-cup serving has 200 calories, 5 grams of fat, and a whopping 13 grams of sugar—and that's before you add anything to it, such as yogurt or milk.

CUT 50 CALORIES AND 12 GRAMS OF SUGAR

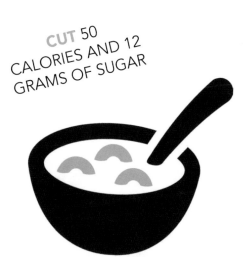

steel-cut oatmeal

## BROTH-BASED SOUP INSTEAD OF CREAM

I admit it, there is nothing better than a cup of tomato soup on a cold day, but with many packing 500 calories per serving, a simple switch to broth can save you 350 calories and still give you the warm fuzzies. Hearty up your soup by adding chunks of veggies or grilled chicken.

*SAVE 350 CALORIES*

*broth-based soup* ↗

*CUT FAT BY 30% AND TRIM 100 CALORIES*

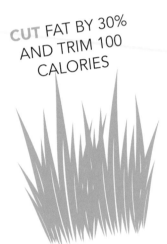

## GRASS-FED STEAK INSTEAD OF STEAK

Not only is the taste out of this world, but grass-fed steak has almost 100 fewer calories and 30 percent less fat per serving than regular steak. Plus, the fat is the "good stuff" and higher in omega-3s—similar to the healthy fats found in seafood.

← *grass-fed steak*

## HUMMUS INSTEAD OF MAYO ON SANDWICHES

Check it out: 2 tablespoons of Sabra hummus is under 60 calories, whereas 1 tablespoon of mayo is 90 calories. But the polar opposite comparisons don't stop there. Mayo is mainly a mixture of oil, and the fat content tops 10 grams per serving. Hummus is not only tasty, but with 8 grams of protein and 7 grams of fiber per serving, it will also make you feel fuller longer!

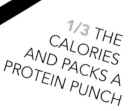

*hummus on sandwich* ↗

*1/3 THE CALORIES AND PACKS A PROTEIN PUNCH*

## KALE CHIPS INSTEAD OF POTATO CHIPS

Hello, life-changer! 1½ cups of kale chips is just 84 calories, while the same amount of potato chips will set you back more than 200 calories. Plus, kale is a "superfood"—one serving meets your entire daily requirement of vitamins A and C, plus it packs calcium and folic acid. Making these chips is so simple: Place the kale on a cookie sheet, spray with olive oil, bake at 350 degrees for about 20 minutes, lightly dust with sea salt, and TA-DA! Amazing!

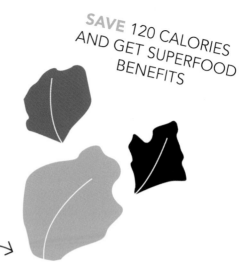

SAVE 120 CALORIES AND GET SUPERFOOD BENEFITS

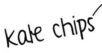

Kale chips

## OLIVE OIL INSTEAD OF BUTTER

This is proof that not all fats are created equal. While butter is a big source of the fats that clog arteries (saturated fat), olive oil has healthy unsaturated fats. It also promotes higher levels of the satiety hormone serotonin, which prevents overeating.

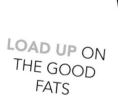

LOAD UP ON THE GOOD FATS

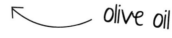

olive oil

## 20-MINUTE EASY, HEALTHY RECIPES

Now that we have our painless swaps down, it's time to talk healthy eating in a flash.

Have you ever searched online for healthy recipes and after about step 20 said to yourself, "*This* is why I don't eat healthy!"?

The truth is, for healthy eating to be doable and sustainable for a family, it has to be easy. And I am talking *quick*.

These CoreCamper.com recipes are a hit with my family and all are fairly simple. That means zero cooking skills required. It also means you can get your family involved in preparing these recipes. Just like how we bring our kids out to "help" us with yard work, in hopes that one day these skills will be transferable—healthy eating and cooking are no different. You have to do it to get it!

*Eating clean feels amazing*

# **CORECAMPER** NO-BAKE PROTEIN BALLS

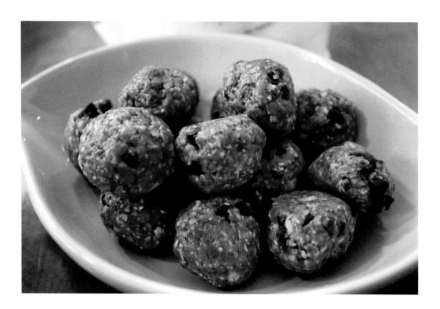

## INGREDIENTS

⅓ cup natural peanut butter

¼ cup honey

1 scoop chocolate whey protein powder

3 Tbsp. ground flaxseed

3 Tbsp. dark chocolate chips

## DIRECTIONS

Mix all ingredients together in a large bowl. Roll into 10 balls (about one heaping tablespoon per serving).

Refrigerate to firm up balls, overnight for best results. Enjoy!

## **CORECAMPER** TURKEY, LETTUCE & HUMMUS WRAPS

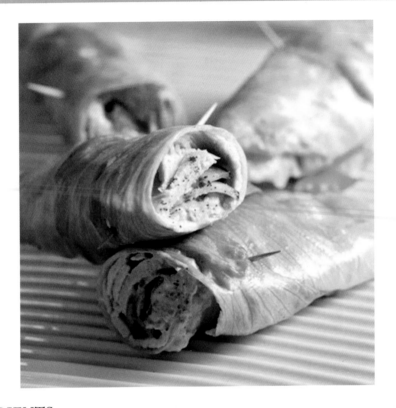

## INGREDIENTS

4 leaves iceberg lettuce

4 slices roast turkey

½ cucumber, sliced

2 Tbsp. hummus

sprinkle of paprika

## DIRECTIONS

Top a lettuce leaf with a slice of turkey, cucumber, hummus, and paprika. Then, as if it were a sandwich, wrap it up with another piece of lettuce.

Repeat with the remaining ingredients.

# CORECAMPER HUMMUS ROASTED VEGGIE PIZZA

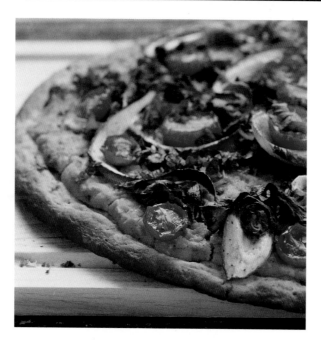

## INGREDIENTS

handful of your favorite veggies (try spinach, tomatoes, and zucchini)

1 Tbsp. olive oil

1 garlic clove, minced

salt and pepper, to taste

1 soft tortilla shell

hummus

low-fat goat cheese

## DIRECTIONS

Roast veggies for about 20 minutes at 350 degrees with the olive oil, garlic, salt, and pepper.

Top your favorite type of tortilla with hummus, add the roasted veggies and some goat cheese, and then bake for 10 minutes at 350 degrees. Slice and enjoy!

# **CORECAMPER** ZUCCHINI PIZZA BOATS

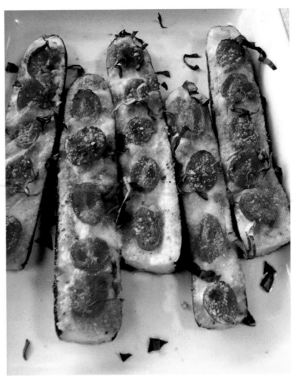

## INGREDIENTS

    3 zucchinis, sliced in
       1-inch slices lengthwise

    natural spaghetti sauce

    chopped turkey pepperoni

    shredded low-fat mozzarella cheese

    basil, for seasoning

## DIRECTIONS

Preheat the oven to 450 degrees.

Wash each zucchini thoroughly. Cut off the ends and cut lengthwise in 1-inch thick long slices.

Place the zucchini boats on a cookie sheet lined with parchment paper.

Smear natural spaghetti sauce on boats. Add sparingly the chopped turkey pepperoni and then cheese. Sprinkle with basil.

Bake for 15 minutes.

# **CORECAMPER** QUINOA BURRITO BITES

## INGREDIENTS

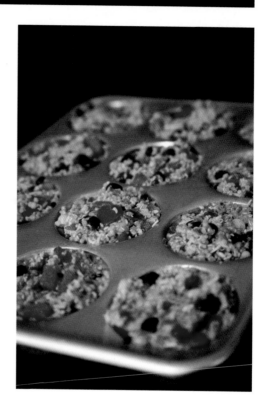

1 cup uncooked quinoa

1 can black beans, rinsed and drained

3 Roma tomatoes, diced

½ red bell pepper, diced

½ cup frozen corn

3 large eggs

1 cup shredded cheddar cheese

2 tsp. minced garlic

½ cup fresh cilantro

1 cup Sabra salsa (plus extra for dipping)

## DIRECTIONS

*Prep:* Follow this step for a faster recipe. Place the uncooked quinoa and two cups water in a covered pot. Bring to a boil, and then simmer for 15 to 20 minutes or until the quinoa is tender. Allow to cool for 10 minutes.

Preheat oven to 350 degrees.

Mix together all ingredients in a large mixing bowl (save some salsa for dipping).

Distribute mixture into a greased muffin tin, filling each cup to the top (about two heaping tablespoons each), and press down gently with the back of a spoon to compact.

Bake for 25 to 30 minutes. Cool for 10 minutes before removing from the pan. Serve warm with salsa for dipping.

Makes 18 muffins.

## **CORECAMPER** ROASTED CAULIFLOWER DIP

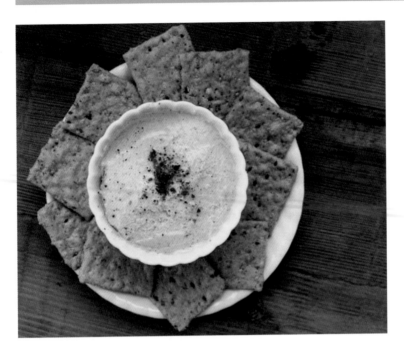

SAVE CALORIES AND FALL IN LOVE WITH THE TASTE. THIS DIP WILL BE A GO-TO RECIPE FOR YOU

## INGREDIENTS

1 head cauliflower (2 lbs.), cut into florets

2 Tbsp. extra virgin olive oil

¼ tsp. whole cumin seed

coarse salt

red pepper flakes

1 cup low-fat plain yogurt

1 Tbsp. lemon juice

## DIRECTIONS

Heat oven to 425 degrees. On a rimmed baking sheet, drizzle cauliflower with oil, and sprinkle with cumin. Season with salt and red pepper flakes. Roast, stirring once, until golden brown and tender, about 25 minutes. Let cool.

In a food processor, puree cauliflower with yogurt and lemon juice.

I eat
healthy
to fuel
my body

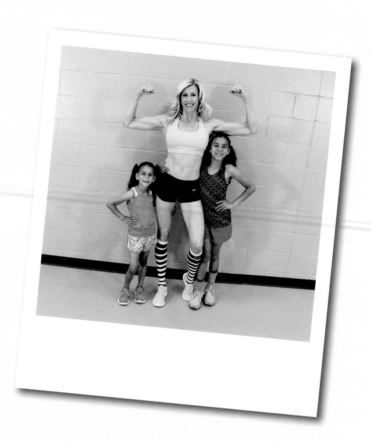

CHILD OBESITY CAUSES MANY TO THROW THEIR HANDS IN THE AIR AND HOPE THEIR KIDS WILL "GROW OUT OF IT." **BUT THERE ARE STEPS YOU CAN TAKE!**

# CHAPTERTHREE
## Kids in Motion

When we were children, our parents had many of the same worries for us as we have for our children. But rising childhood obesity rates is a relatively new concern for parents. It is not easily rectified, especially if the parents are struggling with the same weight issues as their children.

Children are considered obese when their body mass index (a measure of weight in relation to height) exceeds that of 95 percent of their peers of the same age and sex. According to the CDC (Centers of Disease Control) the rate of obesity in children ages six to eleven increased from 6.5 to 19.6 percent from 1980 to 2008. This translates to a tripling of the nation's childhood obesity rate.[1]

This obesity problem doesn't just magically go away after age eleven either. Between 16 to 33 percent of adolescents are now obese—one in three adolescents.

So what can we do as parents? It is a struggle for many that causes them to throw their hands in the air and hope their kids will "grow out of it." But there are steps you can take!

## MAKE FITNESS A FAMILY VALUE

Remember when you were pregnant with your first child and had a lot of free time to ponder, "How will we raise our kids?" In our minds or in discussions with our spouses, many prospective parents talk about how they plan to handle discipline, household expectations, sports, religion, family time, and more. But what about taking care of your body? I find that sometimes this topic doesn't make the cut, even when it really should be one of the star players. Here is how you do it, even if your "babies" are walking around, going through puberty, and moody!

### Model the Behavior

According to Reuters Health, kids who grow up in a household with smokers are three times more likely to also light up and become smokers.[2] Dr. Darren Mays of Georgetown University also did a study showing that teens whose parents were regular smokers were three to four times more likely to smoke.[3] Why am I mentioning this? Because it truly is proof that consistent and disciplined behavior is learned and modeled. The good news is that statistics are actually the same for households where kids grow up with active parents! When you move and make fitness and health a priority in your household, beginning with you, your kids will follow. It may not seem like it, but they are watching and emulating you.

### Use Power Words

I cringe when I hear parents say (often in front of their kids), "She needs to trim down a little bit." By referring to your kids as "Skinny Minnie," "Skin and Bones," "Skinny," "Tiny," and so on, you may be sending them the message that being skinny is a good thing. I even heard a mother recently in a kid's clothing store tell her preteen daughter, "Oh, get those shorts! Your legs look really skinny in them!"

In my household, we don't do skinny. We do strong. How do we do that? As parents, we use those words not only for our kids, but also for us. You see, a lot of these body image issues your kids struggle with are absorbed as they participate in the environment around themselves, which means that many of their attitudes about food, health, fitness, and body strength are extensions of how you feel about you. When children grow up seeing their parent strive for strength, it puts them in a more positive space than having a parent who is always talking about how they need to lose weight to look good. Call your child *strong*!

When your son wakes up in the morning: "Well, good morning, Strong Tyler! Are you ready to conquer the day?!"

After your daughter's soccer game: "You looked so strong during your soccer game, Leah—I am so proud of you for working so hard!"

When someone gives you a compliment: "Thank you! I have been working hard, and I feel strong and amazing."

Words matter and become your inner dialogue. Use them wisely!

### Keep Healthy Foods in the House

I have had this conversation with clients many times. They express concern for their kid's weight issues, and I ask about their nutrition. Many times, parents tell me they "just won't eat" healthy foods. That's when I ask them when their child started doing his or her own grocery shopping.

You see, as parents, we have a lot of battles. We fight some, and we have to let some go.

Toothpaste smeared on the counter after you told them to not do that? Let it go.

The eye roll that you saw her give as she walked up the stairs? Let it go.

The shorts he wants to wear that clearly don't match his shirt? Let it go.

What he or she puts in his or her body? FIGHT FOR IT.

If you are going to hold your ground on one thing as a parent, your children's health and safety are paramount. Yes, that means they might gripe and moan about the healthy foods.

They may even boycott it, sticking their noses in the air and vowing never to eat again. But trust me. They will get hungry. When your back is turned, they will try it. And even though they may not ever admit to you, they will begin to develop a taste for healthy foods if that is what they are offered. Healthy can be tasty, and it is your job as a parent to stick to your guns on this issue.

"No one else eats like this!" may be a whine you will hear.

Your response could be, "We are a healthy family and believe in feeding our bodies good fuel."

Get your kids involved with healthy cooking and the grocery shopping, and teach them how to pack a healthy lunch. These are skills and values they will take with them for years to come.

### Don't Reward with Food

Have you ever offered to get a child a treat if they behave the whole time you are shopping? Or they get an A on a test and their reward is pizza and ice cream? Hey, no shaming here. We have all been there and done that, but it is also something you should be mindful of. Kids who get "treated" with unhealthy rewards grow up to be adults who also "treat" themselves the same way. Don't make unhealthy food synonymous with a job well done. "Treat" them with a trip to the zoo, their favorite movie, an afternoon alone with you, or a play date with their best friend.

### Make Fitness Fun

I should have made this the number one point because it is so important. We often are master salespeople to our kids. "Let's go have some fun at Grandma's today!" sounds a lot better than, "Come on kids, we have to go see Grandma and try not to break anything," right?!

Fitness is no different. I often encourage parents to not only work out with their kids but also keep it playful, short, and silly. Laughing and some healthy competition are a must!

Below is what I call the "Boredom Burner" for kids. It is a great way to get moving, especially on a day where you glance over and see them on a device, watching a cartoon, or being sedentary for long periods of time. Kids just don't "go out and play" as much as they used to, so here is a way to get their heart rates up, bodies moving, and having fun.

This is just a 10-minute workout! Perform each exercise for 40 seconds with a 20-second rest, and then go through this list twice.

# **FROG** JUMPS

Sound effects aren't necessary, but they are highly recommend! Get in a low "froggie" position, knees bent, and hands on the ground. Hop around, trying to get as high as you can! Perform for 40 seconds with a 20 second rest.

STEP**1**

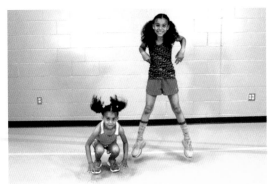

STEP**2**

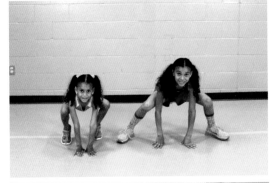

STEP**3**

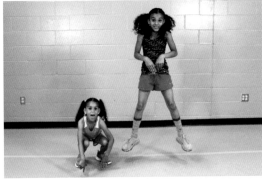

# BEAR CRAWLS

My kids love to try to scare me with this one! Get in a low, all-fours position, knees not touching the ground. Crawl all over the room, staying low like a bear—and growl as loud as you can!

Perform for 40 seconds with a 20 second rest.

STEP**1**

STEP**2**

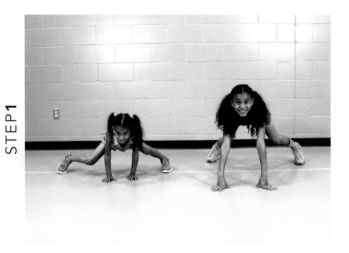

# INCHWORM

Stand tall, with your legs straight and knees unlocked. Place your hands on the ground and walk them out to a straight-arm plank position, keeping legs straight the entire time. Add a pushup at the bottom (optional) and then "inchworm" back up. Perform for 40 seconds with a 20-second rest.

STEP 1

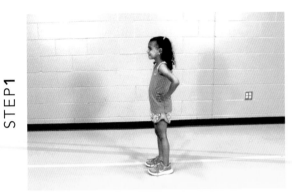

STEP 2

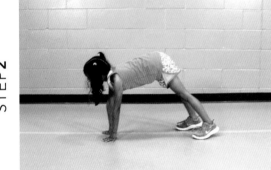

STEP 3

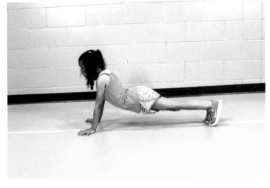

# **FURRY FRIEND** TOSS

My kids love this one because they can also incorporate their favorite stuffed animal friend! They can also use a basketball. Squat low and toss the stuffed animal in the air. Run and try to catch it before it hits the ground! Perform for 40 seconds with a 20 second rest.

STEP**3**
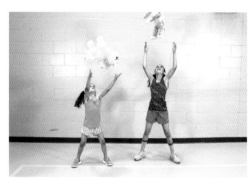

STEP**1**
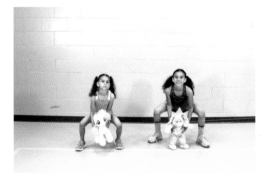

STEP**4**
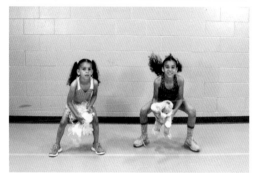

STEP**2**
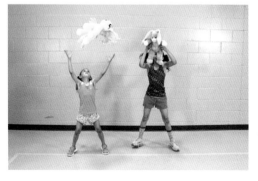

STEP**5**
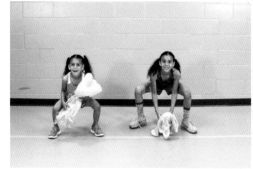

What kid doesn't like an exercise with the word *burp* in it? (Tee-hee!) Place hands on ground (in "froggie" position), jump feet back, and drop to belly. Jump back up with feet by hands. Then jump in the air, reaching as high as you can. Perform for 40 seconds with a 20 second rest.

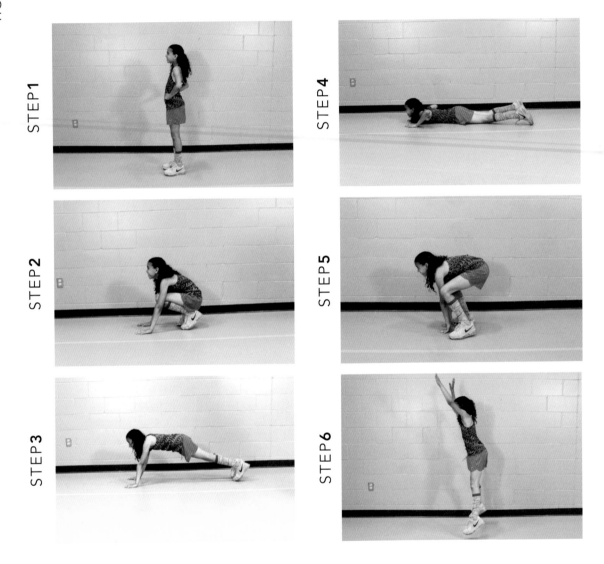

STEP**1**

STEP**2**

STEP**3**

STEP**4**

STEP**5**

STEP**6**

# BURPEES

This is the only body I have, and I will treat it accordingly

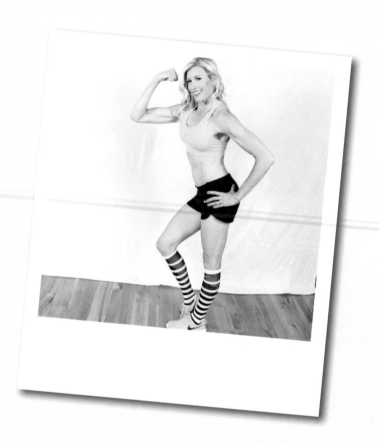

RESEARCH SHOWS THAT 98 PERCENT OF
**DIETS DON'T WORK LONG TERM!**

# CHAPTERFOUR
## Why Diets Don't Work—and What Does!

When someone tells me they are on a diet, my response is always the same. Research shows that 98 percent of diets don't work long term, and even in my business, I have yet to meet the 2 percent they have worked for. And an even more sad fact is that in the United States, research shows that by ten years old, 80 percent of young girls have been put on a "diet."[1]

## SO WHY DON'T THEY WORK?

Whether it was fat-free, no-carb, or all-meat, chances are you have been on a diet and subsequently realized you couldn't keep it up long-term. What I don't like about the word *diet* (I call it the "Dirty D" word) is that it puts you in a negative place. It is synonymous with depriving yourself from foods you love, unrealistic expectations, overly restrictive eating, extra financial costs, complicated "rules," and inconvenient maintenance requirements.

## MY TOP 3 REASONS TO DUMP THE DIET

### 1. *They are detrimental to your metabolism.*

Eating a very low-calorie diet can be extremely harmful to your body's metabolism. If you dip too low in your calorie intake, your body simply compensates by decreasing your overall metabolic rate, which can ultimately hinder your weight-loss goals. Your body decreases its metabolic rate to compensate for this lower calorie level and then turns to lean muscle for energy. This decrease in overall lean body mass lowers your metabolic rate even further as muscle acts as your own personal fat incinerator.

When your body receives too few calories, the minute you go off the low-calorie diet, your body celebrates by putting the pounds right back on.

What to do instead: Aim for about ten to eleven calories per pound of body weight per day. Make sure you are not consuming "empty calories" such as processed foods and sweets.

### 2. *Diets socially alienate you.*

Have you ever been on a diet and avoided a social outing because it was too tempting to eat and attending might derail your diet? Not only do diets deprive you physically, but they can also cause you to isolate yourself from social situations you once enjoyed. I often see this with clients who say they skip getting together with friends because they can't be "good." I call this "Disordered Eating"—creating unhealthy habits that affect not only your body but also your social life, mood, relationships, and more.

What to do instead: A healthy relationship with food means you allow yourself to love it, just with moderation. Split your favorite dish with a friend or don't be afraid to ask the chef to prepare your meal with less oil and no butter. Choose healthier alternatives. Have fun!

### 3. *You can't keep it up long term.*

I recently had dinner with a friend who was entering everything she ate in an app to track her calories, almost obsessively, to the point where she wasn't stopping to just enjoy her meal. Although some of these nutrition-tracking apps are a great idea initially (they help you to educate yourself on proper nutritional values of your favorite foods and appropriate portion sizes), are you really going to be using this app your entire life? When you are measuring food, obsessively tracking, and counting every calorie, you are making eating a job, and you most likely won't maintain that tedious chore long term.

What to do instead: Change your relationship with food. Look at your food as important fuel to keep your body "running" throughout the day. Our bodies are amazing machines that need premium fuel. When you stop having a combative relationship with food and learn to really appreciate it as fuel, you "get" what clean eating is all about.

## SO YOU DUMPED THE DIET, NOW WHAT?

### *Create a Nutritional Game Plan (notice I didn't use the "Dirty D" word?!).*

We often share with our CoreCamper.com clients that by redefining their relationship with food, they will also have better results from their workouts. I tell them, "Abs are made in the kitchen," and that is the truth! Even the most disciplined exercisers need to eat clean in order to see the real results they want—both in their energy levels and muscle definition. Think of clean eating as 70 percent of your success; effective exercise gets to take credit for 30 percent.

Here are some simple Nutritional Game Plan rules to follow:

### *Eat five to six mini-meals per day, or every two to three hours. Eat on a consistent schedule!*

By eating consistently throughout the day (every two to three hours) you will maintain your energy levels by maintaining consistent blood sugar levels. This will aid you in minimizing cravings and making unplanned or poor food choices. Also, by maintaining consistent energy levels, you are more prone to move more, which will reward your weight loss efforts with a calorie-burning boost. Conversely, individuals who eat infrequently tend to eat much larger meals because they are generally much hungrier. By the time they do eat, they make unwise food choices because their body's drive for survival by feeding is pushing them to consume high fat and high calorie feedings at that time. Think of yourself as a hunter and gatherer—eat, burn, eat, burn—you get the idea.

### *Make breakfast the largest meal of the day and dinner the leanest.*

"I had coffee and toast for breakfast" is a sentence I often hear. That's like putting two dollars in your gas tank in the morning to drive around town all day. Doesn't make much sense, does it? By making breakfast your heartiest meal of the day, you are "filling your tank" with clean fuel to get your metabolism jump-started, energy levels high, and your day started. Take your typical size of a breakfast and dinner and swap them. Most Americans eat a hearty dinner and a small breakfast when really we need the "fuel" at the start of our day. Make your dinner your smallest meal of the day because you are more sedentary and will not have the opportunity to burn off that meal.

### *Consume at least a half gram of protein per pound of body weight each day.*

Protein is key because it's what builds and maintains muscle. Why do we need muscle? It is the most efficient and hardworking tissue we have. It burns calories while we sit and watch TV (well done, muscle!). Many women are reaching only half of their recommended daily protein quota. When they tweak the protein in their diet, they are shocked at the results they see—more muscle definition, a leaner body, and increased strength. It is generally recommended that if you are trying to gain and maintain lean muscle, you should aim for a half gram of protein per pound of body weight per day. So if you weigh 140 pounds, 70 grams of protein per day is your goal.

### *Consume approximately ten to eleven calories per pound of body weight each day.*

I touched on this earlier, but it's important to include in the Nutritional Game Plan. Don't obsessively count these calories, but as you get started, be mindful of your calories. If you weigh 140 pounds, that would be roughly 1400 to 1540 calories per day. Remember, this is a benchmark—not a number to be obsessed over! After a few weeks, you will be eating your 5 to 6 mini-meals in smaller portions and find that you don't need to count calories as your body burns food as fuel.

*Drink at least a half ounce of water per pound of body weight each day.*

This is important. Water is essential for our skin, metabolism, and organs. I find it helpful to start the day with a bottle of water and just put a check mark on it each time I fill it up and drink the bottle. Again, if you weigh 140 pounds, aim for 70 ounces of water per day, and make sure you are aware of the nearest restrooms! At the end of the day, your bottle will be covered with check marks, and you will feel proud of reaching your goal!

*Limit your carbs in the evening.*

Protein builds muscle; carbohydrates provide energy. Many of us load up on carbohydrates (breads, pastas, and so on) in the evening for "comfort food" or traditional dinners. But when you really think about it, doesn't it make more sense to eat your carbs when you really need them? Consume carbs in the morning before a busy day, throughout the day as you are busy running around with the kids, or before your workout. In the evening when we are sedentary, we do not need extra energy like we do in the beginning of the day. Focus more on eating protein a few hours before bed, and get ready to feed those muscles while you dream the night away!

*Allow one "cheat day" per week.*

Whenever I meet new clients and tell them they can have a "cheat day," they go crazy the first one. Then they email me and tell me after six days of eating clean, they paid for that cheat meal with a stomachache. But cheating is important—not only does it allow you to still enjoy your favorite indulgences (mine is birthday cake!), but research shows it also helps you reset or "shock" your metabolism after a week of clean eating. I encourage people to use their cheat day wisely, focus on smaller portions, and really notice how that food makes them feel versus the "clean fuel" they consume during the week. It is eye-opening!

## SO NOW THAT YOU KNOW YOU SHOULD'T DIET, WHAT SHOULD YOU EAT?

As you read this Nutritional Game Plan, I want you to go back to my car analogy. It's as simple as this: Think of your body as the most valuable vehicle you could ever own. This amazing, one-of-a-kind, irreplaceable car has a very small gas tank that must be filled every two to three hours in order for it to function.

As you read each meal option, remember that you are changing your view of food. Food is fuel that is necessary and important. You would never put sugar or junk in the world's most valuable car, now would you? Don't do the same with your body.

Let's take a trip!

## BREAKFAST OPTIONS

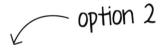
option 1

- **1 PIECE OF EZEKIAL BREAD WITH SCRAMBLED EGG WHITES (½ CUP SCRAMBLED) AND 2 SLICES OF AVOCADO (SEASON WITH PEPPER)**

- **1 CUP OF GREEK YOGURT**

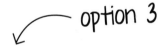
option 2

- **1 CUP OF GREEK YOGURT MIXED WITH ¾ CUP OF KASHI GOLEAN CRISP! CEREAL**

- **1 BANANA**

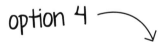
option 3

- **¾ CUP COOKED STEEL-CUT OATS WITH 2 TABLESPOONS FRESH BLUE-BERRIES (SEASON WITH CINNAMON)**

- **PROTEIN SHAKE**

option 4

- **2 WHOLE GRAIN WAFFLES WITH FRESH SLICED STRAWBERRIES**

- **EGG WHITE OMELET IN A MUG: PUT ½ CUP EGG WHITES IN A MUG, SEASON WITH PEPPER. MICROWAVE FOR APPROXIMATELY 2 MINUTES.**

## SNACK OPTIONS

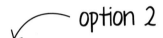
option 1

- 2 TABLESPOONS SABRA GUACAMOLE WITH 10 STACY'S ALL-NATURAL PITA CHIPS

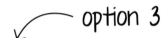
option 2

- 1 PIECE OF STRING CHEESE WITH 2 TABLESPOONS ALMONDS

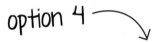
option 3

- 1 RICE CAKE SMEARED WITH 1 TABLESPOON NATURAL PEANUT BUTTER

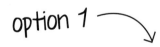
option 4

- 1 APPLE, SLICED. DIP IN 2 TABLESPOONS NATURAL PEANUT OR NUT BUTTER.

## LUNCH OPTIONS

option 1

- TURKEY SANDWICH ON WHOLE GRAIN PITA: USE HUMMUS (2 TABLE-SPOONS) INSTEAD OF MAYO AND ADD DARK GREEN LETTUCE AND 1 SLICE OF SWISS CHEESE

- 1 APPLE

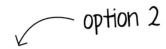

option 2

- **1 GRILLED CHICKEN BREAST (4 OUNCES) WITH ½ CUP BAKED SWEET POTATO, SPRINKLED WITH CINNAMON**

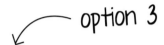

option 3

- **GRILLED CHEESE (SWISS) ON EZEKIAL BREAD. ADD 2 SLICES OF AVOCADO WITH SLICED TOMATO**

- **¾ CUP RED GRAPES**

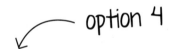

option 4

- **HOMEMADE CHICKEN SALAD: CANNED CHICKEN, ½ CUP GREEK YOGURT, HANDFUL OF CRANBERRIES, AND A HANDFUL OF WALNUTS. ENJOY ON A WHOLE GRAIN ROLL OR PIECE OF EZEKIAL BREAD**

- **½ CUP DARK BERRIES**

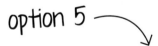

option 5

- **FLATBREAD MARGHERITA PIZZA: WHOLE GRAIN FLATBREAD, SMEAR WITH NATURAL MARINARA SAUCE, SPRINKLE WITH BASIL AND LOW SODIUM SALT, ADD DICED TOMATOES AND A PINCH OF LIGHT CHEESE AND CHOPPED KALE. BAKE AT 400 DEGREES FOR APPROXIMATELY 15 MINUTES.**

## MORE SNACK OPTIONS

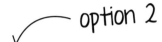
*option 1*

- SLICE A CUCUMBER IN HALF LENGTHWISE, SMEAR WITH HUMMUS, AND ADD TURKEY SLICES. PERFECT CUCUMBER SANDWICH.

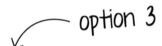
*option 2*

- 2 TABLESPOONS SABRA HUMMUS WITH 1 CUP SUGAR SNAP PEAS

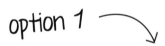
*option 3*

- 1 CUP NATURAL APPLESAUCE WITH DICED APPLES ADDED AND CINNAMON SPRINKLED

## DINNER OPTIONS

*option 1*

- MEAT OF YOUR CHOICE: 4-OUNCE CHICKEN BREAST, FISH, OR LEAN RED MEAT. GRILL, BAKE, OR BROIL.

- 1 CUP STEAMED VEGETABLES OF YOUR CHOICE—SMALL DARK LEAFY GREEN SALAD WITH OIL AND VINEGAR DRESSING

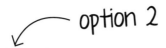

- **HEALTHY CHICKEN CORDON BLEU—(POUND 4-OUNCE CHICKEN FLAT. PLACE PIECE OF SWISS CHEESE ON TOP AND ROLL UP. SECURE WITH TOOTHPICK. DIP IN EGG WHITES AND THEN WHOLE GRAIN CRUMBS. BAKE AT 350 DEGREES FOR 40 MINUTES)**

- **PAIR WITH VEGETABLES OR DARK LEAFY GREEN SALAD**

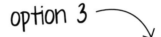

- **4-OUNCE GRILLED SIRLOIN STEAK**

- **10 ASPARAGUS SPEARS (PUT ON A COOKIE SHEET, DRIZZLE WITH OLIVE OIL, BAKE AT 400 DEGREES FOR 20 MINUTES)**

## BEFORE BED OPTIONS

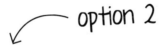

- **PROTEIN SHAKE**

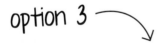

- **½ CUP GRAPES BLENDED WITH ½ CUP OF GREEK YOGURT**

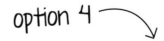

- **30 PISTACHIOS**

- **DARK CHOCOLATE (3 POSTAGE-STAMP SIZED SQUARES)**

- **CUP OF GREEN TEA**

# PREP, PREP, PREP

Now that you know what to eat, it's time to let you in on my little secret: the key to healthy eating is meal prepping.

The biggest benefit of prepping is that it will set you up for success. With busy lives, crazy schedules, and hunger sneaking up on you—you may reach for food that is not part of your healthy-eating initiative. Prepping really saves my nutrition week and takes just about one hour per week.

I typically do my prep on Sunday because that's the day our family naturally falls into "prep mode" for the week. My daughter does her homework, I plan out my TV segments for the week, we make school lunches, we finish laundry—and we prepare our food.

Invest in some good-quality plastic containers and portion out your meals. I usually keep the meals for the following two days in the refrigerator and then freeze the rest if needed (meats).

For the frozen meals, take them out of the freezer and allow them to defrost in the fridge the night before. Then heat them up the next day (whether it be in the microwave or on the stovetop).

Here are some examples of items I prep for the week and portion out into plastic containers. I do this for the entire family so if the kids or my husband are hungry and are on limited time, they can grab one of these meals and eat it within a couple of minutes—and not ask me, "Mom, what can I eat?"

## Proteins

Chicken breast (grilled and baked), ground turkey, lean red meat, and hard-boiled eggs are good sources of protein.

I freeze not only preprepped 4-ounce meat portions but also diced meat. This is perfect for soft tacos, salads, flatbread pizzas, and more.

## Grains

Brown rice, quinoa, and whole grain pasta are excellent sources of grain.

Prep tip: While still warm, toss with 1 to 3 teaspoons of olive oil to prevent stickiness and maintain the flavor.

### Vegetables

Grilled or baked asparagus spears, steamed broccoli, cauliflower, brussels sprouts, spinach, sweet potatoes, green beans, and zucchini are easily accessible vegetables.

### Fruits

Dice up and portion out your fruit.

Prep tip: With fruit ripening, you may need to do the fruit prep portion twice a week instead of just once. Also try sprinkling the fruit with some lemon juice. The citric acid prevents browning and keeps fruit fresh.

### Salads

I often like to have pre-portioned dark leafy green salads. Stock them with diced cucumber, peppers, chickpeas, or some of your other favorites to hearty it up.

## SOME OTHER PREP TIPS

Plan what you are going to prep before you go to the grocery store. Be strategic in your shopping and don't deviate from your list. You are on a mission to be organized, healthy, and economical. Don't fall for the marketing gimmicks thrown at you at every turn in the grocery store.

Track how much money you are saving when you meal-prep. I find this is a huge motivator for families to stick to this healthy eating gameplay of being prepared. You will be shocked at how your grocery bill lowers when you take thirty seconds to tear up your own head of lettuce as opposed to buying a package of mixed greens or a prepared deli salad!

Put a small amount of water in vegetable containers you are storing after prepping. This will keep them fresher and help them hold their flavor.

Wash and portion your fruits and vegetables right when you get home from the store. This can be time consuming and tedious at times, so do it right away. Wash in a clean sink of water with 1 tablespoon vinegar. Soak for 10 to 15 minutes and then rinse. Your produce will taste amazing. With vegetables, the most important part is to cut them up. Sure, we all would love to add that amazing red pepper to our salad—but when running out of time, those nutrient-rich vegetables often get skipped. By having them diced, sliced, and bagged, you are more apt to incorporate this fibrous goodness into your daily meals. Fruit is excellent to portion out per serving. If you have ever sat in front of the TV and demolished a bowl of grapes, you can empathize with me. Those 1-cup-sized portions are ideal and make for organized snacks the entire family can grab and take on the go!

When heating up frozen preprepped meat, put it in a skillet or covered microwaveable bowl and spray with olive oil.

Pre-portion snacks too, such as nuts, berries, and more. That way you can grab them on-the-go.

I will not
"treat myself"
with food

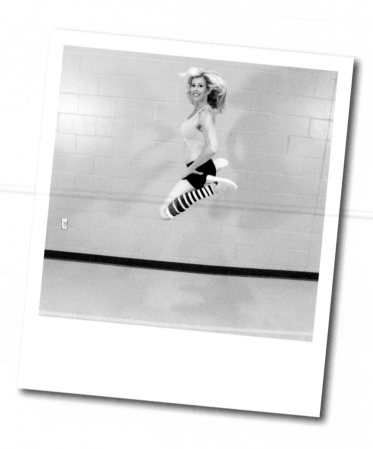

COMPARE THE SUGAR CONTENT OF YOUR FAVORITE FRUIT JUICE WITH YOUR FAVORITE SODA, AND YOU'LL BE MORTIFIED THAT **NO ONE HAS EVER WARNED YOU BEFORE!**

# CHAPTER FIVE

## Elevate Your Snack IQ

Elevating your "Snack IQ" for you and your family is one of the best investments you can make in your health.

The "snack" is a relatively new phenomenon. As a kid, do you remember there being much more in your pantry than maybe some canned soup and spaghetti noodles? Now when I help clients overhaul their pantry, I open the doors to see they have fallen for every "healthy" marketing gimmick: "high fiber," "low fat," "lean," and anything that looks natural.

I call this the Big Business of Health. Companies claim that foods are "healthy" without too much accountability.

Snacking continues to increase in our country and now accounts for more than 25 percent of today's average calorie intake versus less than 5 percent in the 1970s.[1]

Here is another thing to pay attention to: 50 percent of these snack calories come from beverages. We are being marketed to not only in the *food* sections of grocery stores, but also through drinks. Sure, some already look unhealthy (blue in color with cartoon writing on the bottle), but also beware of the "healthy" drinks that are really bottles of sugar and calories. These drinks are usually packaged to look natural, healthy, and expensive—and they are expensive. Most cost upwards of five dollars per bottle, but they include more calories in one serving than our breakfast. Compare the sugar content of your favorite fruit juice with your favorite soda, and you'll be mortified that no one has ever warned you before!

The FDA guidelines for making relative claims are as follows[2]:

## "LIGHT"

*(1) A food representative of the type of food bearing the claim (average value of top three brands or representative value from valid data base), and (2) Similar food (potato chips for potato chips).*

## REAL TALK

When a food is labeled "light," it simply has to have fewer calories than the top three national "non-light" brands. Are you feeling better about thinking "light" means healthy? Me neither.

## "REDUCED" AND "ADDED" (OR "EXTRA," "PLUS," "FORTIFIED," AND "ENRICHED")

*(1) An established regular product or average representative product, and (2) Similar food has at least 25 percent fewer calories per RACC than an appropriate reference food (for meals and main dishes, at least 25 percent fewer calories per 100 grams).*

### REAL TALK

Let's talk real numbers. If a 500-calorie meal has 25 percent less calories, or is "reduced," you are saving only 125 calories.

## "MORE" AND "LESS" (OR "FEWER")

*(1) An established regular product or average representative product, and (2) A dissimilar food in the same product category which may be generally substituted for the labeled food (potato chips for pretzels) or a similar food.*

### REAL TALK

This item can simply have more nutrients or fewer calories and make this claim. Even if it just one gram more or less, it can be used to market to you.

## "HIGH," "RICH IN," OR "EXCELLENT SOURCE OF"

*Contains 20 percent or more of the DV (daily value) per RACC (reference amount customarily consumed). May be used on meals or main dishes to indicate that the product contains a food that meets the definition but may not be used to describe the meal.*

### REAL TALK

Let's say you choose a loaf of bread where each piece contains 2 grams of fiber. To meet this claim and for a company to market a product as "high in fiber," it would only have to have 2.4 grams of fiber. Chances are you are paying more for this "healthier" version, which really is not a significantly improved choice.

## "GOOD SOURCE," "CONTAINS," OR "PROVIDES"

*This is 10 to 19 percent of the DV per RACC. These terms may be used on meals or main dishes to indicate that the product contains a food that meets the definition (has 10 to 19 percent of the DV per RACC) but may not be used to describe the meal.*

## REAL TALK

If you buy a protein bar that is marketed as "provides protein to fuel your day!", this bar only has to have 10 percent more protein than an average breakfast bar. So if a two-dollar box of granola bars has 8 grams of protein per bar, the six-dollar box of protein bars in the health section only has to have 8.8 grams of protein per bar to be marketed as a healthier option.

## "MORE," "FORTIFIED," "ENRICHED," "ADDED," "EXTRA," OR "PLUS"

*This is 10 percent or more of the DV per RACC than an appropriate reference food. May only be used for vitamins, minerals, protein, dietary fiber, and potassium.*

## REAL TALK

Many foods are marketed with the perception that they are healthy by simply using the words *fortified* or *more* in a vague sense. But as consumers who are looking for a healthier option, we tend to fall for this tactic hook, line, and sinker. A box of cereal with "more" fiber only has to have 10 percent more to make this claim. Impressive? No. Will it make a difference in your overall health? Probably not.

## "LEAN"

*Seafood or game meat products qualify as "lean" when they contain less than 10 grams total fat, 4.5 grams or less saturated fat, and less than 95 milligrams cholesterol per RACC and per 100 grams (for meals and main dishes, meets criteria per 100 grams and per labeled serving). On mixed dishes not measurable with a cup (as defined in 21 CFR 101.12[b] in table 2) that contain less than 8 grams total fat, 3.5 grams or less saturated fat, and less than 80 milligrams cholesterol per RACC.*

## REAL TALK

The "lean" claim is a fairly new one and is more specific than other claims. If you are buying "lean" meat, it must contain less than 10 grams fat per 4.5 grams saturated fat. But be aware that there are different levels of "lean." Read the labels and don't be afraid to put them side by side in the store. It's a great way to learn and educate yourself in this confusing world of health lingo!

## "FIBER" CLAIMS

*If a fiber claim is made and the food is not low in total fat, then the label must disclose the level of total fat per labeled serving.*

## REAL TALK

Look at the nutritional value as a whole. For example, if a manufacturer increased the fiber so they could market the product as such—did they also add other "unhealthy" ingredients to make the product taste better?

I mention all of the above text because you can see for a company to claim a product is healthy, in many cases it only needs 10 percent of your recommended daily value of those nutrients. *10 percent?* You mean I just paid double for a "healthy" product for a mere 10 percent increase in the nutritional value?

Educating yourself on how to choose healthy snacks will not only benefit your health but also save you money. With prepackaged "health-conscious" foods, the quantities are small, the processing is aplenty, and the prices are high. It's all about marketing, because food producers, after all, want your money. It keeps them in business to sell you something.

So how do you snack sensibly?

Picture yourself at about 3:00 p.m. on a Monday afternoon. It isn't time for dinner yet. Your energy is nosediving, and you really want to reach for a candy bar and call it a day. But then that little voice perks up and says, "Hey, weren't we trying to eat healthy and not fall for empty calories?" Oh yeah.

One of the biggest nutrition struggles for people is snacking. What are sensible options? How much can you eat? And what will keep you full until your next meal?

My suggestion is to choose snacks that contain 200 calories or less, keeping in mind that the purpose of the snack is merely to "refuel" you until you get to your next meal.

When eating five or six mini-meals a day, these under-200-calorie snacks truly become mini-mini-meals. They are not intended to be as substantial as breakfast, lunch, or dinner, but they should not be considered a throwaway mini-meal. Here is a quick go-to guide for healthy snacks:

## 40 FILLING, NUTRITIONALLY-DENSE, AND TASTY SNACKS UNDER 200 CALORIES

1. 1 banana with 10 almonds

2. 1 slice Ezekial bread topped with one ounce of cream cheese spread

3. 1 cup Greek yogurt with 1 teaspoon drizzled honey

4. 1 square dark chocolate and 1 ounce dried cranberries

5. 1 cup blueberries

6. 1 cup grapes

7. 1 cup orange slices sprinkled with cinnamon

8. 10 Stacy's Pita Chips with 2 tablespoons Sabra hummus

9. 1 ounce smoked salmon on a ½ whole grain English muffin, smeared with light cream cheese

10. 2 rice cakes smeared with 2 tablespoons Sabra hummus

11. 1 chocolate rice cake smeared with natural nut butter and 10 mini dark chocolate chips on top

12. 2 pieces of low-sodium sliced turkey, wrapped around a piece of string cheese

13. 1 cup sliced cucumbers with 2 tablespoons Greek yogurt (plain, squeezed with lemon)

14. 1 cup sugar snap peas with 2 tablespoons Sabra hummus or Greek yogurt dip

15. 2 large hard-boiled eggs

16. 1 cup unsweetened applesauce, sprinkled with cinnamon and 4 pecans on top

17. ½ baked sweet potato, sprinkled with cinnamon

18. 1 cup cottage cheese with pineapple chunks

19. 1 piece of Laughing Cow light cheese with 8 whole grain crackers

20. 1 pear and one piece of string cheese

21. 1 slice Ezekial bread smeared with natural peanut butter and low-sugar jelly

22. 1 cup raw veggies and 2 tablespoons Bolthouse Farms salad dressing

23. ½ cup canned chicken or tuna and 8 whole grain crackers

24. 1 cup whole grain tortilla chips and 3 tablespoons salsa

25. whole grain English muffin (½), smeared with light cream cheese and topped with apple slices

26. 40 pistachios

27. ½ apple (sliced) with 2 tablespoons natural peanut butter

28. 2 cups of air-popped popcorn

29. ¼ cup almonds or cashews

30. English muffin pizza: spread natural pasta sauce, a pinch of mozzarella, and a sprinkle of basil.

31. 8 ounces of fat-free chocolate milk

32. ¾ cup Kashi GoLean cereal and ½ cup cashew milk

33. 1 tablespoons natural peanut butter spread on 2 celery stalks

34. 1 ounce whole wheat pretzels, dipped in 1 teaspoon spicy mustard

35. 1 cup steel-cut oats, sprinkled with cinnamon

36. 3 ounces turkey jerky

37. 2 cups cherries

38. 1 ounce sunflower seeds

39. 8 dried figs

40. 1 cup vanilla Greek yogurt mixed with 1 scoop chocolate protein powder

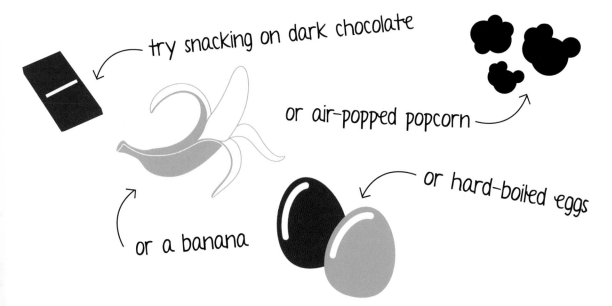

try snacking on dark chocolate

or air-popped popcorn

or hard-boiled eggs

or a banana

# PORTION SIZES 101

When you are a healthy eater, learning to "eyeball" portion sizes will be one of the most valuable skills you can learn. Have you ever met a person who measures their food on a scale? Chances are they are (*a*) no fun to be around and (*b*) not doing it the next time you see them. Measuring and obsessing are short-term, unhealthy habits that only lead to you eventually throwing your hands in the air out of frustration.

One of my favorite ways to really make portion sizes relatable is to compare portions to everyday objects. It works, it sticks, and it's fun. But first, how much should you be having? Let's break it down. The United States Department of Agriculture (USDA) recommends you have the following daily. Keep in mind, with our CoreCamper Nutritional Game Plan, you are spreading these servings out over your five to six mini-meals per day.

## *USDA Daily Recommendations*

breads and grains: 6–11 servings

fruits: 2–4 servings

vegetables: 3–5 servings

dairy: 2–3 servings

protein foods: 2–3 servings

fats, oils, and sweets: use sparingly

Okay, so now that we know how much we should be eating, you may have a question that you think you should know the answer to. How much is in a serving? You would be surprised how many people whisper this question to me, almost sheepishly, because they think everyone knows but them. Not true, and I am going to make it easy for you.

## *How to "Eyeball" a Portion*

breads and grains: 1 serving = 1 compact disc (CD)

fruits: 1 serving = 1 tennis ball

vegetables: 1 serving = 1 lightbulb

dairy: 1 serving = 2 dice or 1 cup milk

protein: 1 serving = a deck of cards

fats, oils, and sweets = no more than two thumbprints

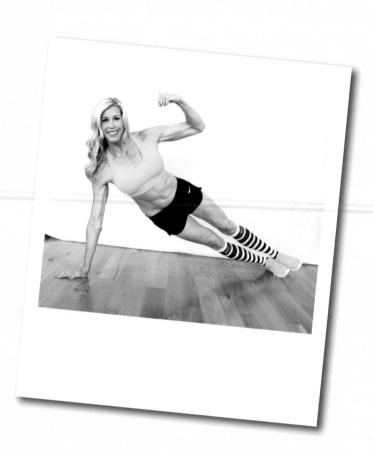

YOU ALMOST NEED A MAP TO NAVIGATE YOUR WAY AROUND
**THE GROCERY STORE!**

# CHAPTERSIX
## Grocery Store Navigation

Is it just me, or have you noticed that grocery stores have become massive? You almost need a map to navigate your way around, and it truly is a marketers' paradise. Endcaps with exciting health claims, samples galore with pushy tasters, buzzwords everywhere you look like "healthy," "high fiber," "rich in antioxidants," and of course my favorite words: "on sale!" It is hard enough to go to the store and stick to your list. Bring your kids with you and it becomes a total free for all.

One of the biggest downfalls people have when trying to eat healthier is bringing foods in their home that derail them. I often tell my clients, "If it comes in a box, chances are your body will resemble a box." We are in the age of processed foods, and they are everywhere. It's no wonder we are all craving convenience. We are out of time most days, and those marketing and advertising companies are just getting better at hitting our sweet spot.

## SIX CONVINCING REASONS TO AVOID PROCESSED FOODS

### 1. *Processed foods are usually loaded with added sugar and high-fructose corn syrup.*

It is well known that sugar, when consumed in excess, is seriously harmful. Sugar is also "empty" calories. It has no essential nutrients and can have devastating effects on your metabolism that go way beyond the empty calories. Excessive sugar can lead to insulin resistance, high triglycerides, increased levels of the harmful cholesterol, and increased fat accumulation in the liver and abdominal cavity. It also is associated with some of the world's leading killers, including heart disease, diabetes, obesity, and cancer.

### 2. *High-sugar foods lead to overconsumption.*

Processed foods are engineered, and they are so engineered that they are incredibly "rewarding" to the brain. Our bodies are smart and are composed of complicated mechanisms that regulate energy balance (that is simply how much you eat and how much you burn). This energy balance was what made hunters and gatherers lean with efficient bodies. But with the rise in these engineered foods, the reward value of foods can bypass the innate defense mechanism and make us start eating much more than we need. I call this the "no off switch."

### 3. *Processed foods are loaded with artificial ingredients.*

Want to study a different language? Read a processed food label. The reason it all is so foreign is because many of the ingredients aren't actual food. They are artificial chemicals that are added for various purposes.

Highly processed foods often contain the following:
- preservatives: chemicals that prevent the food from rotting
- colorants: chemicals that are used to give the food a specific color
- flavor enhancers: chemicals that give the food a particular flavor
- texturants: chemicals that give food a particular texture

Sounds yummy, right? Here's the kicker: keep in mind that processed foods can contain dozens of additional chemicals that aren't even listed on the label.

For example, an "artificial flavor" is a proprietary blend, and manufacturers don't have to disclose exactly what it means. These artificial flavors are usually a combination of chemicals and could mean that there are ten or more additional chemicals that are blended in to give a specific flavor or texture.

### 4. *Processed foods can be addicting.*

The hyper-rewarding makeup of processed foods can activate the same areas in the brain as drugs of abuse like cocaine. That's scary. In fact, adults and kids can literally become addicted to processed foods and the intense dopamine release that occurs in the brain when these foods are consumed. I am a big believer that "food addiction" is as serious of a problem as drugs and alcohol because people literally can't stop. The cravings are real, not only psychologically but physiologically as well.

### 5. *Processed foods are full of refined carbohydrates.*

Refined simple carbohydrates are quickly broken down in the digestive tract, leading to rapid spikes in blood sugar and insulin levels. This leads to carbohydrate cravings just a few hours later when your blood sugar plummets. This has been called "crashing and burning." You feel your energy level drop dramatically, which tempts you to refuel with unhealthy processed foods again. It is a vicious cycle.

### 6. *Processed foods require less energy and time to metabolize.*

In order to have a longer shelf life, most of the fiber and nutrients have been taken out of processed foods, making them easier to chew and digest. Remember the "You Can't Eat Just One" slogan? This rings true more than you know with processed foods. By eating nonprocessed foods, you are burning twice the amount of calories to metabolize that meal than you would with a boxed meal.

## READING LABELS 101

Before I tell you what to look for, first I want to drop some label knowledge on you.

How do you read a label, and what in the world are we even looking for? Who measures their food in grams?

The American Heart Association recommends the following:

**FAT** People should consume 500 to 700 calories from fat each day, somewhere between 56 to 78 grams daily (or 25 to 35 percent of your total daily calories). It is also recommended that you limit your saturated fat intake to less than 16 grams and keep unhealthy trans fats to less than two grams per day.[1]

**SUGAR** It's recommended that women eat 100 calories from added sugars each day—that's about 5 percent of their daily diet, or about 20 grams daily. This is equivalent to about 6 teaspoons of sugar. You may think that seems generous, but consider this—a can of soda will get you to this quota in about 3 gulps. The AHA's new guidelines don't include sugar found naturally in fruits, vegetables, whole grains, or milk. "Added sugars" are sugars that are added to food in processing and also to sugars and syrups used to make foods or drinks.[2]

**SALT** The recommended daily intake of salt is 1500 milligrams to 2300 milligrams per day, which is only about a teaspoon of salt. Are you thinking to yourself, *I don't put salt on my food*? Well, not so fast. Check a frozen "healthy" prepackaged meal, which will reach that quota in one sitting.[3]

So now that you are armed with the information, it's time to hit the grocery store. What do you do first? Make a list. Would you ever go to a business meeting without grabbing your notes? Treat the trip to the store as a strategic plan you are going to try to stick to. I also get my kids involved. I give them mini lists of items I know they can easily find and bring back to me, such as plain Greek yogurt, egg whites, apples, whole grain bread. Once we find something we like, it falls into our Nutritional Game Plan and budget. My kids know the brands we choose, and I show them why. Am I trying to win the "Parent of the Year Award"? No. But I am trying to teach them how to navigate a store for health, because before I know it, they will be shopping on their own (*sniff, sniff*).

## MAKE A MAP

Mental maps count here too. I am going to save you tons of time at the grocery store with this tip: Shop on the perimeter of the store 80 percent of the time. When you avoid the center, you avoid the prepackaged temptations. Hit the produce, meat, dairy and grains instead. I also acknowledge you will have to pass the bakery on the perimeter. Stop there only on special occasions!

Here are some must-haves from the grocery store:

### *Pantry Foods*

* cereal (we like Kashi GoLean Crisp! and KIND)
* steel-cut oatmeal
* whole wheat crackers
* brown rice
* whole wheat pasta
* organic tomato sauce (check the ingredients—you want a sauce made with only tomatoes, olive oil, and spices—no corn syrup or sugar added)
* canned diced or whole peeled tomatoes
* canned tuna, chicken, or salmon packed in water
* low-sodium canned beans (chickpeas, pinto, black, kidney, and so on)
* basic seasonings and sauces: Mrs. Dash Salt-Free Seasoning, balsamic vinegar, red wine vinegar, Ken Davis 2 Carb low-sugar BBQ Sauce, Boathouse Farms salad dressing
* healthy oils like extra virgin olive oil, canola oil, and nonfat cooking spray
* dark chocolate
* an assortment of green teas
* dried fruit
* fruit leathers
* avocados

### *Refrigerator Foods*

* fruits and veggies (including staples of apples, oranges, lemons, lettuce, tomatoes, cucumbers, kale, dark leafy greens, asparagus, zucchini, and onions)
* nonfat or low-fat milk
* nonfat or low-fat Greek yogurt or cottage cheese
* egg whites and eggs

- nuts
- natural peanut butter and nut butters
- Sabra hummus and Greek yogurt dip
- Sabra salsa and guacamole
- low-fat cheese (reduced-fat cheddar, part-skim mozzarella, or reduced-fat string cheese sticks)
- low-sodium and lean turkey bacon
- whole wheat English muffins
- whole grain or flax flatbread
- Ezekial bread
- quinoa
- butter alternative (nonhydrogenated and without trans fats)
- mustard

### Freezer Foods
- frozen vegetables (get the option with no cheese, no butter sauce, and so on)
- frozen fruit (raspberries, strawberries, blueberries)
- ground turkey
- skinless chicken breasts
- lean red meat
- salmon
- frozen Greek yogurt ice cream

## "ORGANIC" TIP

If you are on a tight budget and can't afford the organic options, that is okay. But if you can, try to buy organic when purchasing peaches, nectarines, strawberries, celery, bell peppers, lettuce, pears, imported grapes, cherries, potatoes, and apples.

### Foods That Are Not as Important to Buy Organic

Pineapples, mangoes, kiwis, bananas, papayas, blueberries, watermelon, onions, avocados, sweet corn, sweet peas, asparagus, cabbage, broccoli, and eggplant may not be quite as critical to purchase organic because the outer layer (where pesticides and chemicals sit) is removed prior to eating.

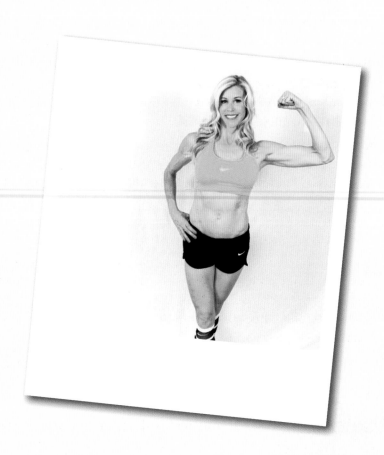

JOIN THE
"DROPKICK THE SCALE" CRUSADE!

# CHAPTERSEVEN
## The Great Weight Debate

From weight loss shows with extreme numbers to our neighbor lady bragging that she got down to her high school weight, we are programmed to associate losing weight with being healthy and strong. Nothing can be further from the truth, and for the past fifteen years, I feel like I have been on a "Dropkick the Scale" crusade.

Turns out, talking people into not weighing themselves is harder than it would seem. Why is that? Let's start with the doctor's office. It's where we go to get our health checked when we aren't feeling so great, right? So why does the nurse throw us on the scale the minute we walk into the office? I get it. If you suddenly have an extreme weight gain or loss since your last visit, this could be a clue to an underlying health problem. But why are the health experts still using weight as a determinant of body health?

If you are an active person, your body weight can be one of the most misleading and frustrating numbers in your life. First, let me answer the question I get all the time: "Does muscle weigh more than fat?" Answer: no. A pound of fat weighs one pound. A pound of muscle also weighs one pound. But muscle *is* more dense than fat. In fact, a pound of fat takes up four times more space than a pound of muscle. Still not convinced?

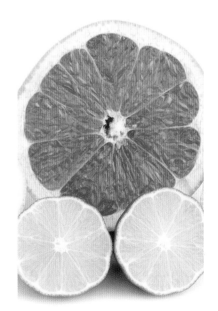

Picture this: One pound of fat is the size of a large grapefruit. One pound of muscle is the size of a small lime.

This means the more lean muscle you gain, the smaller you will appear, but oftentimes your weight won't budge—in fact, it might (*gasp!*) go up.

But what about BMI (body mass index)? BMI is a value derived from the weight and height of an individual. So should we pay attention to it? Here is the short answer: body fat is a much more accurate determinant of success.

I compare it to feeling like you have a broken arm. Calculating your BMI is like having the doctor just feel your arm to see if it is broken. But if you focus on body fat and not your BMI, it is like having an X-ray to see what's really going on inside your arm. In fact, when you put most professional athletes on the BMI scale, they are classified as obese. Flash a picture of a guy with six-pack abs in your head. He can't be obese! He looks pretty fit to me!

So what can you do to really measure your success when you are involved in a workout and healthy eating program? Here are my top four tips:

## 1. DROPKICK THE SCALE

Believe it or not, I have had clients sneak and weigh themselves even when I told them not to. Sounds crazy, but as women, we are so tied to a number. We grew up hearing our moms either complain about "the number" or try to get to "the number." Now that you know you are barking up the wrong tree, it is time to say good-bye to the scale.

## 2. BUY A MEASURING TAPE

Measuring yourself will prove the fact that muscle is more dense than fat. As you are gaining lean muscle, you will feel your body shrinking and getting more toned.

These numbers also have significance far beyond how you look. According to the National Institute of Health[1] and a study done by the American Cancer Society[2] with 48,500 men and 56, 343 women, an increased waist circumference measurement could lead to increased risk for type 2 diabetes, hypertension, and cardiovascular disease. The recommendation is no more than thirty-five inches for women and no more than forty inches for men. Even slight decreases in waist circumference can greatly reduce your risk of developing these life-threatening diseases and will also reflect progress in your fitness program.

After many years of being a trainer, here is where I have found are the best places to measure:

**Chest:** Place the measuring tape just below bust, where your bra line is, keeping measuring tape parallel to floor as you wrap around. This is a great measurement spot for upper abs.

**Abs:** I like to measure right at the belly button line because this is the true "girth" of your abs. Wrap tape around your body, keeping parallel to the floor.

**Dominant leg:** Wrap the measuring tape around your dominant leg at the largest part of your thigh, keeping measuring tape parallel to floor

**Dominant arm:** Choose your most used arm and wrap the tape around the largest part of your bicep. Arm is not flexed but relaxed.

**Hips:** Wrap measuring tape around the largest part of your butt and hips, keeping parallel to the ground.

**Neck:** Sounds crazy right? But have you ever noticed when people get fit, you can see it in their face? This is also a great measurement to show that you can look strong all over! Wrap tape around your neck, as if you were measuring for a dress shirt.

### When should you measure?

I tell my clients to measure every four weeks. This gives you enough time to see success, but also little enough time to get yourself back on track if you feel you are not following your exercise and nutrition plan as well as you should be.

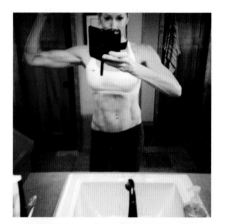

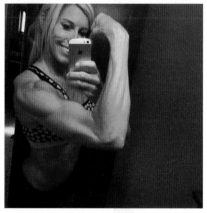

## 3. MEASURE YOUR BODY FAT

This isn't as easy as having your husband or a friend help you with measurements, but it is a good tracking tool to have. You can purchase fat calipers online inexpensively, and they come with complete directions. Calipers simply measure body fat through the thickness of folds of skin on the body, giving you a percentage ratio of muscle to fat. You can also ask a trainer at your gym to caliper measure your body fat every four to six months. This takes minutes and can really be a great motivating tool.

The "athlete" range for women is 14 to 20 percent, "fitness" range is 21 to 24 percent, "average" range is 25 to 31 percent, and "obese" range is 32-plus percent.

## 4. TAKE AN AB SELFIE

This sounds silly, but when you are tracking your success, grab your phone, head to the bathroom mirror, and take a picture! I'm not talking about a picture you can be bribed with if you ever decide to join politics but rather what I like to call an "ab selfie." No one has to see this picture. But sometimes we don't see ourselves objectively. Taking a selfie every four weeks and then putting those pictures side by side can be very eye-opening. You can actually see your progress from the outside and really give yourself some credit. And who knows, one day you may just be brave enough to post it! You go, #StrongGirl!

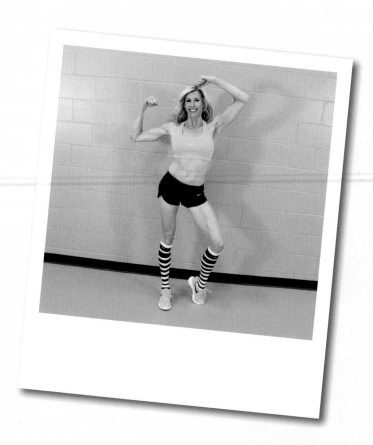

NOT ONLY DOES STAYING ACTIVE HAVE GREAT AESTHETIC
BENEFITS, BUT IT ALSO WILL CARRY YOU THROUGH LIFE
**WITH LESS PAIN, MORE MOBILITY, AND A BETTER ATTITUDE.**

# CHAPTER EIGHT
## If You Rest, You Rust

Have you ever tried to talk with a fifteen-year-old about how the decisions they are making now will affect the rest of their life? If so, how long was the blank stare? The point is often missed because it is not an immediate issue and teenagers have trouble imagining themselves as "old."

Believe it or not, I get the same blank stare when I explain the importance of staying active *now* so that your body will thank you when you are seventy, eighty, and beyond.

My grandmother is 103 years old and still lives by herself in the same home my dad grew up in. She has never taken medication or had any major health issues, and she chugs around her neighborhood like a little steam train. Great genes? Maybe. But she also adopted the "if you rest, you rust" philosophy. Not only does continuing to move and staying active have great aesthetic benefits, but it will also carry you through life with less pain, more mobility, and a better attitude.

## "SITTING IS THE NEW SMOKING"

When I do speaking engagements with large companies, I usually start my presentation with this statement. It may sound shocking, but I believe it to be true. In fact, for your heart health—According to the American College of Cardiology and Dr. David Coven, a cardiologist with St. Luke's-Roosevelt Hospital Center in New York, sitting for two hours is the equivalent of having two cigarettes.[1]

A "standing" worker will burn about 1500 calories during an eight-hour shift. A person in a cubicle will burn roughly 500 calories during the same amount of time. That translates into real numbers and explains why people gain sixteen pounds, on average, within eight months of starting sedentary office work. Sixteen pounds?! Now that is something to pay attention to!

## WHAT TO DO?

For those who sit at a desk all day, getting up and moving around may seem like something you don't have time for, but you don't need a lot to get those essential fat-burning enzymes in your body turned back on. Set an alarm on your phone for every one to two hours. When it goes off, take three minutes and get moving. Go walk three flights of stairs.

Go greet a coworker at the other end of the building, walking briskly. Or just stay in your office and do a series of 10 squats, 10 pushups, and 10 lunges consecutively for those 3 minutes. It doesn't take much, but keep moving! Your waistline and heart will thank you.

In this chapter, I also want to dig deeper into why exercise is so important. This has nothing to do with how we'll look in a bathing suit. As we get older, we look for deeper meanings in why we do what we do. We look at friendships as investments instead of going-out partners. We appreciate our parents more and are more forgiving of the past. We allow our kids to be kids because we realize that time of carefree selfishness will be short lived and should be savored.

We also should look at fitness with the same perspective. Yes, short-term benefits are wonderful—but what about the long-term investment we are making in us?

It's important to reflect on why you are taking the time to exercise when you are feeling discouraged. Other benefits of exercise, which have nothing to do with how you look, will give you more reason to keep on keeping on.

## EXERCISE STRENGTHENS RELATIONSHIPS

It's no secret that when we do not feel good about us, we often try to grab those around us and pull them down as well. We don't do it intentionally, but insecurity and depression loves company and can be a downward spiral for many. When you feel better physically, you feel better mentally, and that translates to our friendships, family relationships, and marriages. Often, during a first meeting with a client, I meet someone who is not happy with where they are physically. Not surprisingly, many have an overall negativity that has permeated far beyond a gym. Feeling alienated from those who exacerbate your insecurities, not wanting to get undressed in front of your husband, and succumbing to being jealous of others weaves its way into your life and can be a lonely place.

I love watching people find their strength. My daughters have both had those butterfly kits, where we start with the caterpillars who transform into chrysalides and then, after a couple weeks, become beautiful butterflies. Getting fit is similar to this gradual transformation. When you feel strong and good about you, you are a better wife, mother, friend, sister, and daughter.

## EXERCISE IMPROVES YOUR SEX LIFE

Put the kids to bed and read this section. Exercise can boost the physical intensity and quality of sex simply because it increases your hormone levels. It also increases your blood flow to your entire body, making you feel more alert and ready for a romp. It also is a great stress reliever, leaving you feeling less irritable, more in the mood, and more confident in your own skin. Because, let's face it, when we don't feel good naked, it sometimes is hard to fully embrace an activity that requires it! Cortisol plays a key role as well. Chronic stress takes a toll on your body. You feel the rush of adrenaline without an off switch, leading to an overproduction of cortisol, or the "stress hormone." Cortisol can cause not only weight gain but also heart issues. There are two key ways you can shut off the production of cortisol: exercise and sex!

A study in the *Journal of Sex Research*[2] and the *Journal of Sex Medicine*[3] found that women were more sexually responsive and had improved blood flow and circulation after just twenty minutes of vigorous exercise.

The release of testosterone is also strongly linked to exercise. Testosterone helps to fuel our bodies, both male and female, by improving our libido and helping us look and feel good—two good combinations for a healthy sex life.

We have all heard the phrase, "A confident woman is a sexy woman," and this is true. When you feel good about your body, you also feel more open with your partner.

## EXERCISE MAKES YOU A BETTER MOM

Sound like a far reach to you? Think again. Regular exercise changes not just your body and metabolism but also your mood. Exercise has a unique effect of exhilaration and relaxation at the same time—all while giving you a feeling of being stimulated but balanced and calm at the same time. Exercise also reduces levels of the body's stress hormones, such as adrenaline and cortisol and stimulates the production of endorphins, which are often called the body's natural painkillers and mood elevators. Sounds like a stage set for better parenting, right? Parenting can be one of the most tumultuous roller coaster rides of stress, anxiety, laughter, and frustration. Exercise is the perfect medicine to make you a more patient, calm, and fun parent.

## EXERCISE MAKES YOU A KICK-BUTT GRANNY

No granny panties, memory loss, and crotchety attitudes here. In fact, a recent study done by the *British Journal of Sports Medicine* with seven hundred participants (eighty-six women total, all seventy to eighty years old) proved that exercise improved the size of the brain, when typically aging has the opposite effect. Participants who reported being physically active (defined as working out twice a week for six months) tended to have larger brain volumes of gray and normal white matter. Regular exercise also appeared to protect against the formation of white matter lesions, which are linked to thinking and memory decline.[4]

In aging, exercise also has been shown to have amazing mood and mental health effects. Staying active also equates to staying more alert, social, and engaged with others. This is not only about living longer, but really striving to live better.

## EXERCISE GIVES YOU BETTER SKIN

Of course, exercise provides benefits to our body, but the improved circulation also does wonders for our skin. Increasing blood flow with exercise helps nourish skin cells and keeps them vital. Blood circulating carries oxygen to working cells, keeping you looking vibrant, healthy, and youthful. Don't believe me? Take a photo without makeup before you start a fitness regimen and then four weeks after. You will be amazed at your new "glow."

## EXERCISE MAKES YOU A BETTER EMPLOYEE

Exercise increases discipline, resilience, energy, health, and commitment. I don't know about you, but I would hire someone with these qualities in a heartbeat. Sticking to an exercise program proves not only to yourself but also to those around you that you are reliable and a follow-through person. It also teaches you that failure is okay and how to rebound and get back in the game after a failure. Being able to better manage, accept, and learn from your shortcomings—and those of your team—will only make you a better employee and leader to be around.

## EXERCISE MAKES YOU THE ENERGIZER BUNNY

I often hear people state they can't exercise because they are just too tired. I get it—life is busy, and the thought of putting on our tennis shoes and doing physical activity when we are exhausted seems equivalent to climbing Mount Rushmore. But the truth is, exercise will reenergize you. In fact, a study done at the University of Georgia proved that regular workouts can boost energy levels by 20 percent and decrease fatigue by 65 percent! Even just fifteen to twenty minutes of exercise a day can be the equivalent of three cups of coffee and is a better alternative. So, yawn, get your shoes on, get moving, and be energized.

# I am strong and unique

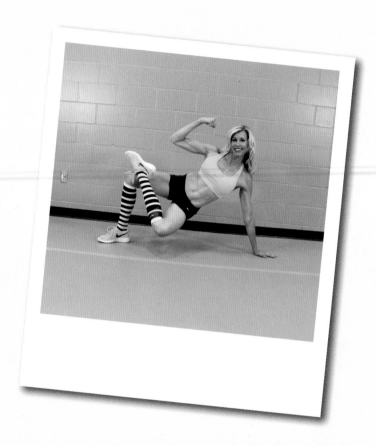

YOU JUST CAN'T SEEM TO MUDDLE THROUGH WHAT'S **FACT OR FICTION WHEN IT COMES TO HEALTH.**

# CHAPTER NINE
## No Such Thing as a "Stupid Question"

I had to include this chapter, and even though it may not be chapter 1, it may be one of the most important chapters. I have been a trainer for years, and when most people have the opportunity to talk to me one on one, they usually begin with, "This may sound like a stupid question, but . . ."

Most of these people are smart, educated, extremely competent people who have been able to get a handle on pretty much everything in life except health and fitness. Isn't that so frustrating? You have worked for an education, built a family, maintained friendships, decorated a house, financed a mortgage, and helped with third-grade math homework. (Is it just me, or is this one the hardest?) But you just can't seem to muddle through what's fact or fiction when it comes to health.

When I get down to where people really are in their health-and-wellness journey, I find that they have created their Wellness Plan through myriad tidbits of resources—a magazine article, their know-it-all neighbor, a Facebook post, Pinterest, a half-hour infomercial when they couldn't sleep one night—and what does this lead to? Complete and utter confusion and misdirection. No wonder so many people give up on this journey before they really figure out it can be a beautiful instead of a frustrating.

Here are some of the "stupid" questions I have received over the years. Let's clarify, cut to the chase, and lay the rumors to rest once and for all.

## 1. IF I DO ENOUGH CRUNCHES, WILL I GET A SIX PACK?

*Answer:* No. In fact, a six pack has nothing to do with crunches. I always tell people that abs are made in the kitchen. The number one thing you need to do is check your nutrition. Switch to mini-meals of real, nonprocessed foods. Also, ensure you are getting enough protein to build *and* maintain that lean muscle. Finally, do effective exercise, such as interval training to help lower your body fat and reveal your six pack. Crunches work about 25 percent of your abs. Try some of the core exercises I show here in this book for better results.

## 2. SHOULD I TAKE A DAY OFF IF I AM SORE?

*Answer:* Get back on the horse. Working out when you are sore will actually help alleviate the soreness and stiffness you may be experiencing from a tough workout. You are feeling DOMS, which is delayed onset muscle soreness. Keep working out and you will find that after a few weeks, that soreness will become less frequent. Not being sore is not a sign of a bad workout—it just means your body is now better prepared for exercise.

## 3. I HAVE ACHES AND PAINS. SHOULD I ICE OR USE HEAT?

*Answer:* First, we have to clarify that there are two basic types of athletic injuries: acute and chronic. "Acute pain" has a rapid onset and is short-lived. "Chronic pain" develops slowly and is persistent and long-lasting.

Acute injuries are sudden, sharp, traumatic injuries that occur immediately (or within hours) and cause pain. Most often they result from some sort of impact or trauma such as a fall, sprain, or collision, and it's pretty obvious what caused the injury.

Acute injuries also cause common signs and symptoms of injury such as pain, tenderness, redness, skin that is warm to the touch, swelling, and inflammation. If you have swelling, you more than likely have an acute injury. Ice is ideal for acute injuries because it reduces the swelling and pain.

Chronic injuries are typically subtle and slow to develop. They sometimes come and go and may cause dull pain or soreness and are often the result of overuse. Heat is ideal for sore, stiff, nagging muscles, or joint pain. You may also use heat therapy before exercise to increase the elasticity of joint connective tissues and to stimulate blood flow. Heat can also help relax tight muscles but should not be used after exercise. Ice is a better choice on a chronic injury post-workout.

## 4. WHY AM I NOT GETTING THE SAME RESULTS WITH RUNNING THAT I USED TO?

*Answer:* Welcome to the plateau. I often see this with people who rely on primarily cardio, such as running, for their main source of exercise. The fact is, doing too much steady-state cardio (such as running, working on the elliptical, and biking) can actually slow your metabolism. It is as basic as your body's survival instincts. Your body adapts to constant training in as little as six weeks. Therefore the body finds it easier to perform and burns fewer calories in the process. Also, bear in mind that when performing steady-state cardio, you only burn extra calories during the exercise. After you've finished, your metabolism returns to normal fairly quickly—that means no afterburn effect we talked about previously in the book. Instead, focus more on metabolic or interval training for better results in less time.

## 5. SHOULD I STOP EATING AT 7:00 P.M. EVERY NIGHT?

*Answer:* I heard this myth on a popular TV show about ten years ago, and it won't die. The truth is it is not really about *when* but *what* you are eating. It is true, the nighttime hours are the time when we are most likely to eat mindlessly and thus overeat. If we find ourselves eating not-so-healthy foods in front of the television during those after-dinner hours, that's a habit that can cause weight problems. I call this mindless eating. You started with a bowl of chips, and then you get into a TV show. Next thing you know, the chips are gone. But eating a healthy mini-meal before bed is actually a good idea. If you restrict food in the evening, you are more than likely to make up for it later. Skipping meals after six will make you feel starved first thing in the morning, and you will probably reach for something unhealthy quickly.

For evening eating, I recommend a protein-rich snack, such as pistachios, protein shakes, egg white omelets, or turkey and string cheese. Stick to your five or six mini-meals a day to keep your insulin levels stabilized, and don't stress about the time on the clock.

## 6. SHOULD I DO A "HOT YOGA" CLASS TO BURN MORE CALORIES?

*Answer:* "Hot Yoga" is one of the hot new fitness trends, no pun intended. Will it make you sweat more? Yes. So will going for a walk in the middle of summer in Arizona. But just because you are sweating more does not mean that you are burning more calories. The elevated calorie burn in a hot yoga class is partly due to the body working hard to cool itself down. A hot room does make for a more challenging workout, but that does not mean it is more effective. Avid participants often report a one to three pound weight loss during class, but this is purely water weight and will return when you rehydrate. We have seen wrestlers do this for years: sweat to drop weight. It works temporarily. You will literally weigh less (the amount of water you sweat out), but the second you rehydrate, you are right back to where you started. Unfortunately no extra calories have been burned and no extra fat has been used for fuel because you are sweating more. Doing these classes to improve flexibility and clear your mind is a better expectation than to see major weight loss results.

## 7. CAN I TURN FAT INTO MUSCLE?

*Answer:* No. They are two different tissues, and one does not magically transform into the other. Muscle is active tissue that burns calories as what I like to call your "personal fat incinerator." When you move, your body will burn more calories, similar to a how a car will burn gas as you travel from point A to point B. Fat, on the other hand, is just a storage of excess energy. The good news is that when you eat clean and exercise, you lose fat and gain lean muscle—but that muscle is not fat that has had a dramatic makeover!

## 8. SHOULD I STRETCH BEFORE MY WORKOUT TO PREVENT INJURY?

*Answer:* Yes, but with *dynamic* stretching, not *static* stretching. Dynamic stretching is stretching with movement. Think of arm swings, slow squats, jogging in place, and marching heels to rear. This type of stretching is emulating the movements you are intending to do with exercise—just not aggressively.

Think of your muscles as hard taffy. You have to slowly start bending that taffy to make it more pliable. If you fold it in half and hold it, that hard taffy would crack, right? Our muscles are no different. After your muscles are warm and pliable, you may proceed with exercise.

Post-workout is when you take advantage of static stretching with those muscles that are warm and pliable like taffy that has been left out in the sun. Exercises such as stretching your arm across your body and holding for 8 seconds and pulling your heel up to your rear and holding for 8 seconds are examples. I often cringe when I am driving and see people next to a trail, preparing for a run and static stretching. Doing this puts you at greater risk of aches, pains, and injuries.

## 9. WILL I GET BULKY IF I LIFT WEIGHTS OR DO TOO MANY SQUATS?

*Answer:* Somebody stop the madness! Excuse my frustration, but this myth just won't die. I don't hear this concern from men too often, but many women express worry over this myth.

Here is the real deal: Without assistance from testosterone-boosting supplements, women cannot achieve extraordinary muscle growth. Because our testosterone is lower, we are not "wired" to get bulky. In fact, it is very difficult, and you have to intentionally be on a highly regimented testosterone supplement program to do so. I am a huge fan of using your own body weight as the best piece of equipment to get a lean, ripped, and functional body. I also find that people tend to perform exercises better using just their own body weight. But if you decide to pick up the weights, don't worry. You will not be ripping out of your shirt and pants anytime soon.

## 10. CAN I JUST BURN FAT IN ONE TARGETED AREA?

*Answer:* Spot training does *not* work. At the end of the day, it all comes down to your overall body fat blanketing those perfectly toned muscles. No matter how many crunches you do, a person with 25 percent body fat will never have abs like someone with 10 percent body fat. Work your body as a unit, utilizing multiple major muscle groups at once for the biggest bang for your buck. Also, keep your nutrition in check. This plays a significant role in seeing results in your "problem areas" as well.

*I will not compare myself to others*

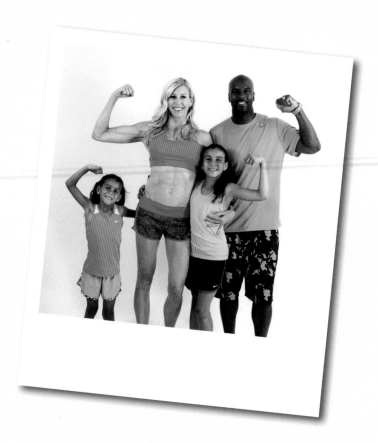

REMEMBER THAT
**THIS IS A PROCESS.**

# CHAPTER TEN
## Closing

During my workouts, I call the final few minutes "the finale," where you begin to pick up the pace and intensity, pushing through as if you are running with your arms spread wide, chest open, and chin up through a finish line tape! I feel the same way about this book.

I have been a trainer and fitness expert for years and have received thousands of questions—many of them the same questions, with different phrasing. It truly has been my dream to write this book, to be a resource to women and families, and to provide a "handbook" of sorts that you can turn to for the "real deal" on health and fitness.

I thank you from the bottom of my heart for taking the time not only to read this book but also to implement some of the strategies I have taught throughout it. Remember that this is a process. Fitness and health means nothing if it does not become your journey—and not something you *have* to do. It all does not have to be done at once. Set small goals. I encourage you to take this journey week by week and, if needed, day by day. Even making the goal to pre-prep your dinners for the next five days or get active as a family starting with five minutes a day is a start. Just remember—you are still lapping everyone on the couch!

Don't take this journey alone. Take it with those you love, because it can truly be meaningful, life-changing, and FUN! I wish you peace, health, laughs, great food, and of course strong abs!

—Ali

I want to live
a long and
healthy life

# #STRONGGIRLS
## FOR LIFE!

"Not only is Ali Holman a fitness expert and motivator, but she is also such an inspiring example of what girls can look up to as a business owner who also puts her family first. She is the definition of #StrongGirl!"

—*Sherry Dopp*

"Being a single parent, working full time, Ali's training philosophy is perfect for me and, to be honest, for anyone! No excuses with her quick workouts, and they have changed my life in a matter of a few months! Ali's meal plans, recipes, and workouts have made me a lifelong follower."

—*Missy Nanoff*

"Ali's motto, 'If you have a body, you *are* an athlete' is truly where all of her advice stems from. She will inspire, motivate, and teach you how to fit fitness into your life!"

—*Heidi Streeter*

"I'm a busy mom of three who loves CoreCamper.com! Ali is the real deal for practical, fun exercise that gives results. The best part is that my kids join me now and we work out together! Ali is a proven expert who practices what she teaches!"

—*Lisa Rudquist*

"I have never liked the shame-game that plays out in the majority of gyms around. The great thing about Ali is she invests in people. She educates them about nutrition and proper form workouts in whatever spectrum (beginner to former athlete) they may fall in. I love the comfort of working out in my own home and the use of simple weights. There is never a day that goes by that I do not feel challenged, empowered, and encouraged by Ali. She is America's diamond in the rough world of fitness."

—*Phil Jones*

"I am a 'math brain' person. I am no-nonsense, work full time, and have three sons and a husband. I like to feel healthy and strong, but with my busy schedule I need the biggest 'bang for my buck.' If you are a person who is always looking at the best ROI on your time invested in working out and getting the best results, Ali is THE ONE AND ONLY."

—*Lori Gherardi*

"Being a stay-at-home mom with three very active girls, I don't have time to go to the gym, nor do I have the money to pay a personal trainer who is really just to pass the time and *maybe* try and help with what my body really needs. I love that Ali shows different levels of exercise I can choose from AND I can get my butt kicked in less than twenty minutes! My family also benefits from her great recipes! All of that together makes me a #StrongGirl and one #StrongMomma!"

—*Mindy Herr*

"Ali gives me everything I need to be a #StrongGirl every day. Not only does she help me stay healthy, but I now also have my son doing the workouts with me. Nothing better than teaching him about daily exercise at a young age and showing him that having a #StrongGirl as a #StrongMom is the model for a #StrongFamily."

—*April Nelson*

"Love Ali's overall message that it's okay for girls to have muscles, embrace fitness, be themselves, not be afraid to show hard work and its lifestyle, and be proud!"

—*Kim Wuebkers*

"#*StrongGirl* means capable, tough, confident, and athletic. Ali Holman helps 'girls' of all ages to become strong girls!"

—*Terrie Allen*

"I love that with Ali I get a brand new workout, and every day I get my butt kicked! Best of all, her workouts are under twenty minutes and I do them at my own time and in the comfort of my own home (or any hotel room around the world for that matter, considering I've 'taken Ali with me" to Aruba, Europe and the Middle East)! I have never, ever felt healthier or stronger than I feel today. Corecamper.com is a no-brainer!"

—*Rania Michelon*

*I will treat
a setback as
a comeback*

# #STRONGGIRLS
## FOR LIFE!

Share your #StrongGirl pics with Ali by tweeting @corecamper on Twitter, posting on Instagram and tagging @corecamper, or posting on Facebook @corecamper.com!

*Ali's canine CoreCampers*

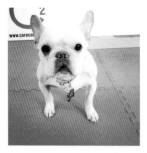
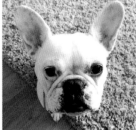
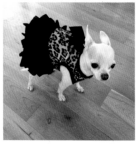
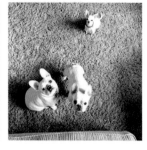
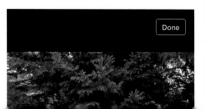

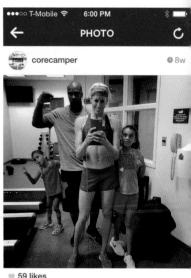

●●●○○ T-Mobile 🔋 6:00 PM 🔋
**PHOTO**

corecamper  8w

🤍 59 likes
corecamper Family #Corecamper #Workout I'm the #Tennessee hotel! 20 mins and we're DONE!

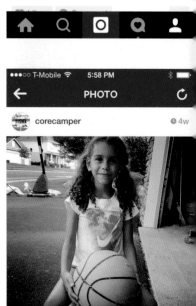

●●●○○ T-Mobile 🔋 5:58 PM 🔋
**PHOTO**

corecamper  4w

🤍 13 likes
corecamper L♥VE #StrongGirl

🤍 Like  💬 Comment  •••

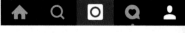
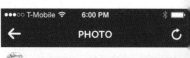

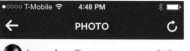

●○○○○ T-Mobile 🔋 4:48 PM 🔋
**PHOTO**

houseofcavalli  45m

Done

●●●○○ T-Mobile 🔋 6:00 PM 🔋
**PHOTO**

corecamper

← **PHOTO** ↻

houseofcavalli   🕑45m

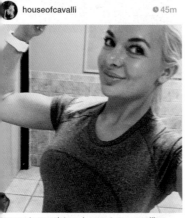

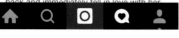

sweatsavvysisters, lumenatorgv, raadling, jkelly9000, beastmode_stazio, vivbambara, vcwrestler125

**houseofcavalli** This ones for @corecamper congrats on your book! I met Ali a few years back and immediately fell in love with her

🏠  🔍  ⬜  💬  👤

← **PHOTO** ↻

corecamper   🕑11w

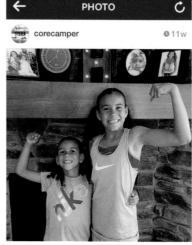

♡ **110 likes**

**corecamper** These two #StrongGirls are coming on @twincitieslive with me today! Please watch AND get the code to get 50 PERCENT OFF our CoreCamper.com online

🏠  🔍  ⬜  💬  👤

**Done**

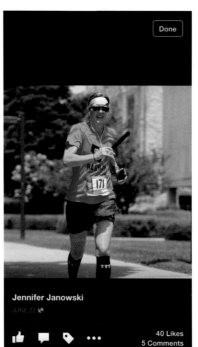

**Jennifer Janowski**
JUNE 22 🌐

👍  💬  🏷  •••        40 Likes
                       5 Comments

←   🔍 Mindy Herr

Mindy Herr
8 minutes ago via Instagram · 👥

A whole new meaning to **#StrongGirl**
@corecamper loving life!!
**#WeFlexonSundays**

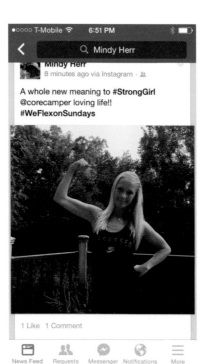

1 Like  1 Comment

📰        👥        💬        🌐        ☰
News Feed  Requests  Messenger  Notifications  More

**Done**

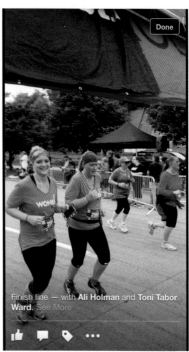

Finish line — with **Ali Holman** and **Toni Tabor Ward**. See More

👍  💬  🏷  •••

← **PHOTO** ↻

corecamper   🕑11w

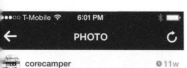

**Done**

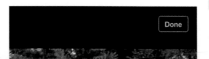

← **PHOTO** ↻

corecamper   🕑5w

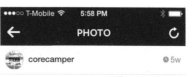

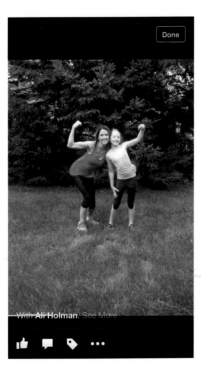

Done

With **Ali Holman**. See More

👍 💬 🏷 •••

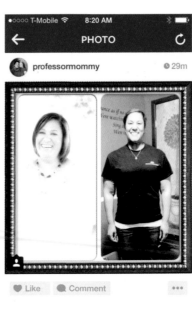

●○○○○ T-Mobile 🕾    8:20 AM    ✻ ▭

←     **PHOTO**     ↻

professormommy     🕑 29m

♡ Like     💬 Comment     •••

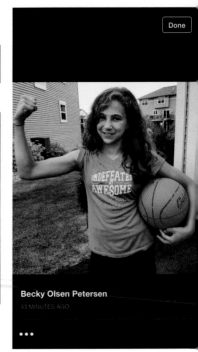

Done

**Becky Olsen Petersen**
43 MINUTES AGO

•••

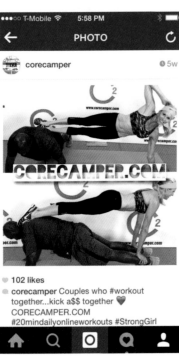

●●○○○ T-Mobile 🕾    5:58 PM    ✻ ▭

←     **PHOTO**     ↻

corecamper     🕑 5w

♡ 102 likes

corecamper Couples who #workout
together...kick a$$ together 🖤
CORECAMPER.COM
#20mindailyonlineworkouts #StrongGirl

🏠 🔍 📷 💬 👤

🏠 🔍 📷 💬 👤

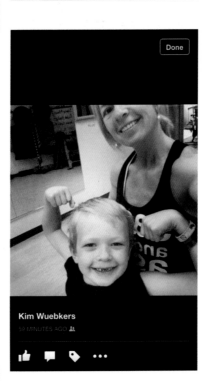

Done

**Kim Wuebkers**
59 MINUTES AGO 👥

👍 💬 🏷 •••

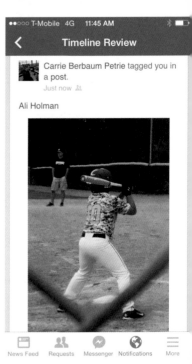

●●○○○ T-Mobile   4G   11:45 AM    ✻ ▭

‹     **Timeline Review**

Carrie Berbaum Petrie tagged you in
a post.
Just now 👥

Ali Holman

🗞 👥 💬 🌐 ☰
News Feed   Requests   Messenger   Notifications   More

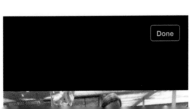

Done

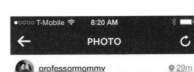

●○○○○ T-Mobile 🕾    8:20 AM    ✻ ▭

←     **PHOTO**     ↻

professormommy     🕑 29m

Done

# What I am doing today will help me in one, ten, and twenty years from now

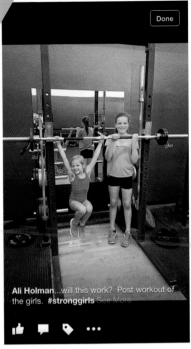

**Ali Holman**...will this work? Post workout of the girls. **#stronggirls** See More

👍 💬 🏷️ ...

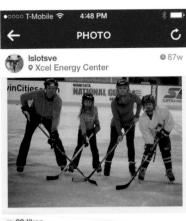

●●○○○ T-Mobile 📶     4:48 PM     ⚹ 📶

←     **PHOTO**     ↻

**lslotsve**     🕐 87w
📍 Xcel Energy Center

💙 **28 likes**
● **lslotsve** We skated on the MN Wild Ice at Xcel Energy tonight- dream come true!
**kmarshall1822** Looks fun
**lslotsve** @corecamper #stronggirls #stronggirl family hockey
**lslotsve** @corecamper #stronggirls #stronggirl
**lslotsve** Family hockey

🏠   🔍   ⊙   💬   👤

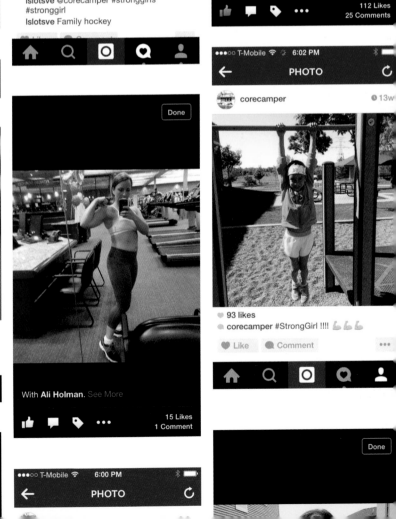

Done

Getting it in with **Christine Hodges, Ali Holman** and Mark Holman. **#chall**... See More

👍 💬 🏷️ ...     **112 Likes**
    25 Comments

●●●○○ T-Mobile 📶     5:58 PM     ⚹ 📶

←     **PHOTO**     ↻

**corecamper**     🕐 4w

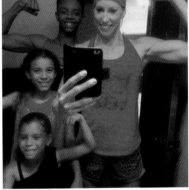

💙 **20 likes**
● **corecamper** We just did 200 push-ups! #fitFam ! #TreyDoesMinnesota

💙 Liked   💬 Comment     ...

🏠   🔍   ⊙   💬   👤

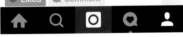

Done

With **Ali Holman.** See More

👍 💬 🏷️ ...     **15 Likes**
    1 Comment

●●●○○ T-Mobile 📶     6:02 PM     ⚹ 📶

←     **PHOTO**     ↻

**corecamper**     🕐 13w

💙 **93 likes**
● **corecamper** #StrongGirl !!!! 💪💪💪

💙 Like   💬 Comment     ...

🏠   🔍   ⊙   💬   👤

●●●○○ T-Mobile 📶     6:00 PM     ⚹ 📶

←     **PHOTO**     ↻

Done

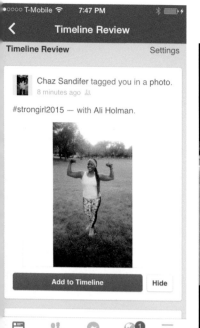

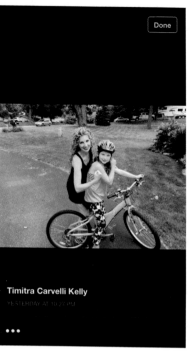

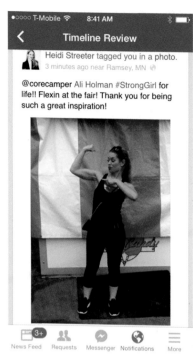

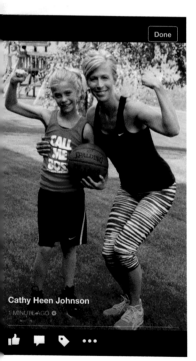

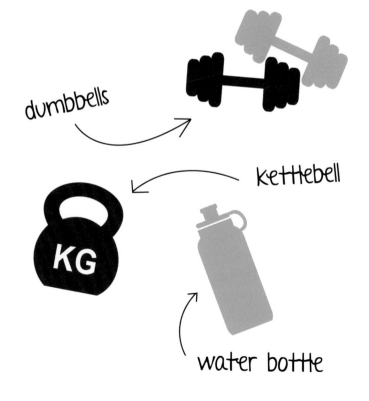

dumbbells

kettlebell

water bottle

# NOTES

## CHAPTER 1

1.  American College of Sports Medicine, "High Intensity Interval Training," accessed June 2013, http://www.acsm.org/docs/brochures/high-intensity-interval-training.pdf?sfvrsn=4.

## CHAPTER 3

1.  Centers for Disease Control and Prevention, "Division of Nutrition, Physical Activity and Obesity," accessed 2011–2014, http://www.cdc.gov/obesity/data/childhood.html; and "Trends in the Prevalence of Extreme Obesity Among U.S. Preschool Aged Children," *Journal of American Medical Association*, accessed December 2012, http://www.cdc.gov/obesity/downloads/jama_highlights_final_data_source_added_011013.pdf.

2.  Reuters Health, "The longer parents smoke, the more likely their kids will too: study," accessed May 13, 2014, http://www.reuters.com/article/2014/05/13/us-teen-smoking-parents-idUSKBN0DT1QV20140513.

3.  Darren Mays, "Children of Nicotene-Addicted Parents More Likely to Become Heavy Smokers," Georgetown University, accessed May 12, 2014, http://gumc.georgetown.edu/news/children-of-nicotine-addicted-parents.

## CHAPTER 4

1.  Common Sense Media, "Children, Teens, Media and Body Image," accessed January 21, 2015, https://www.commonsensemedia.org/research/children-teens-media-and-body-image.

## CHAPTER 5

1.  "Snacking Constitutes 25 Percent of Calories Consumed in U.S.," IFT.org, accessed June 20, 2011, http://www.ift.org/Newsroom/News-Releases/2011/June/20/Snacking-Constitutes-25-Percent-of-Calories-Consumed-in-US.aspx.

2.  "Guidance for Industry: A Food Labeling Guide," FDA.gov, accessed January 2013, http://www.fda.gov/Food/GuidanceRegulation/GuidanceDocumentsRegulatoryInformation/LabelingNutrition/ucm064908.htm.

## CHAPTER 6

1.  American Heart Association, "Know Your Fats," accessed April 29, 2015, http://www.heart.org/HEARTORG/Conditions/Cholesterol/PreventionTreatmentofHighCholesterol/Know-Your-Fats_UCM_305628_Article.jsp.

2. American Heart Association, "Sugars 101," accessed November 2014, http://www.heart.org/HEARTORG/GettingHealthy/NutritionCenter/HealthyEating/Sugar-101_UCM_306024_Article.jsp.

3. American Heart Association, "Shaking the Salt Habit," accessed May 18, 2015, http://www.heart.org/HEARTORG/Conditions/HighBloodPressure/PreventionTreatmentofHighBlood-Pressure/Shaking-the-Salt-Habit_UCM_303241_Article.jsp.

## CHAPTER 7

1. National Institute of Health, "Assessing Your Weight & Health Risk," http://www.nhlbi.nih.gov/health/educational/lose_wt/risk.htm.

2. "Waist Size Matters," Harvard School of Public Health, accessed September 10, 2015, http://www.hsph.harvard.edu/obesity-prevention-source/obesity-definition/abdominal-obesity/.

## CHAPTER 8

1. "Screen-Based Entertainment Time, All-Cause Mortality, and Cardiovascular Events: Population-Based Study With Ongoing Mortality and Hospital Events Follow-Up," accessed April 2011 (study cited by Dr. Coven, Luke's Roosevelt Hospital), http://www.sciencedirect.com/science/article/pii/S0735109710044657.

2. D. C. Frauman, "The relationship between physical exercise, sexual activity, and desire for sexually activity," accessed 1982, *The Journal of Sex Research* 18: 41–6.

3. L. D. Hamilton, A. H. Rellini, and C. M. Meston, "Cortisol, sexual arousal and affect in response to sexual stimuli," accessed 2008, *Journal of Sexual Medicine* 5, no. 9: 2111–8.

4. Lisanne F. ten Brink, et al., "Aerobic exercise increases hippocampal volume in older women with probable mild cognitive impairment: a 6-month randomized controlled trial," *British Journal of Sports Medicine*, accessed October 22, 2013, revised January 15, 2014, http://bjsm.bmj.com/content/early/2014/03/04/bjsports-2013-093184.abstract?sid=ecff0a48-d4fd-4a9d-b34a-156ca915a79e.

# ABOUTTHEAUTHOR

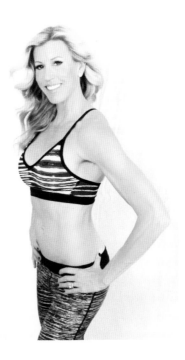

**ALI HOLMAN** has been a national television fitness and wellness expert for over ten years, inspiring people all over the country to fit fitness and health into their busy lives with her "if you have a body, you are an athlete" mantra. As a mom, wife, trainer, television personality, and business owner, Ali's motivation and advice come from a real approach with specific action steps and game plans. She and her husband, Mark, have created CoreCamper.com, an online subscription site that allows you to choose from three daily difficulty levels of new-daily 20-minute online workouts. Ali has created her "smarter, not longer" training method that allows you to never plateau or get bored with your fitness routine. She also gives non-diet weekly Nutritional Game Plans that focus on a real-life way of eating for the whole family.